HERB
Identifier & Handbook

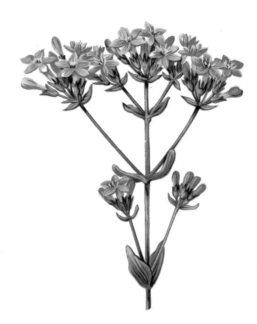

Ingrid Gabriel

Sterling Publishing Co., Inc.   New York

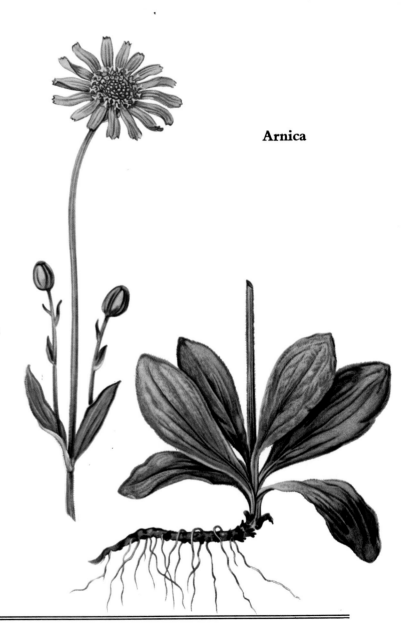

Arnica

All the color illustrations come from *Die Heilkräuterfibel* by
Ernst Gardemin and Hans Weitkamp with the exception of those on
pages 4, 85, and 94, which are by the author. Most of the black-
and-white drawings are by the author, with additional drawings by
Shizu Matsuda

10 9 8 7 6 5 4 3 2 1

Published by Sterling Publishing Company, Inc.
387 Park Avenue South, New York, N.Y. 10016
© 1979 by Sterling Publishing Company
Adapted from the German book *Die farbige
Kräuterfibel* © 1970 by Falken-Verlag
Translated by Manly Bannister. Adapted by E. W. Egan
Distributed in Canada by Sterling Publishing
℅ Canadian Manda Group, P.O. Box 920, Station U
Toronto, Ontario, Canada M8Z 5P9
Distributed in Great Britain and Europe by Cassell PLC
Villiers House, 41/47 Strand, London WC2N 5JE, England
Distributed in Australia by Capricorn Link Ltd.
P.O. Box 665, Lane Cove, NSW 2066
Manufactured in the United States of America
All rights reserved

Sterling ISBN 0-8069-8550-X

CONTENTS

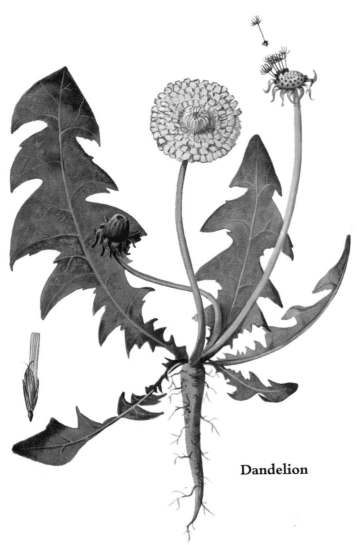

Dandelion

INTRODUCTION

From ancient times to the beginning of the modern era, people of all classes had a comprehensive knowledge of the effect of plants on human beings, medicinally and as foods and seasonings, without having investigated the materials composing them; yet, modern man, except for the skilled specialist in the field, takes a Sunday stroll in the woods without suspecting the treasures surrounding him—usually he does not even know the names of the many herbs growing there. In the past few years, however, not only does the interest of scientists in the healing power of plants appear to have increased, but also many ordinary people are just becoming aware of the priceless service Nature is offering them, if only they knew how to make use of these herbs as simple remedies and as a supplement to their diet.

This handy guide provides a clearly presented introduction to some of the most useful medicinal and culinary plants found nowadays in woods, fields and parks, and many that can be grown in the home garden.

The plants are arranged in alphabetical order, according to their most commonly used names. An illustration accompanies each specific plant. If you are looking for a certain herb, you have only to look up either the English or the Latin name in the index.

Enjoy yourself as you observe the plant world in wood, meadow or garden with this guide book!

MEDICINAL USES

You have been feeling well and then have become ill. Did you know that you can get help from a plant which you normally think of as a garnish for meat dishes—parsley!

In a certain sense, every edible plant is a medicinal plant, for they all serve to normalize the intestinal bacteria and have other beneficial effects on the human system. For example, the effect of lettuce is calming, soporific, antispasmodic; it eases inflammation, cleans, and builds blood. Even a bad case of anemia can be remedied in a short time by a daily dish of raw vegetables, consisting of green lettuce, herbs, carrots, and raw cabbage. At the same time, sugar and all foods prepared with it, as well as white flour, must be avoided.

In one group of plants, the medicinal effect is especially strong, and they are designated as strictly medicinal plants. For a long time, medicinal plants did not stand in particularly good repute, for the world of medicine had discovered chemical preparations that worked a lot more quickly and which appeared to be very advantageous, but which have proved to have harmful side effects. Consequently, modern science has again turned to plants and their medicinal effects, which have been demonstrated over thousands of years of experience, and whose harmful effects are known.

Among the many past advocates of herbal remedies for human illnesses were the Swedish philosopher Albertus Magnus (13th century); the Swiss physician Paracelsus (16th century); Carolus Linnaeus, the Swedish botanist (18th century); and the German priest and healer Sebastian Kneipp (19th century).

Modern pharmacology, however, has not only confirmed old knowledge, but has even been able to discover new uses for some plants, for example, chamomile.

Never evaluate the medicinal elements in plants in terms of quantity. Many a substance that is present only in small traces serves the sole purpose of stimulating the other substances present to be effective. As in homeopathy, it is not always the largest dose that yields the best result.

If you want to enhance the effect of a herb-tea treatment, introduce it to your body along with a suitable diet. Beneficial substances are found in raw or stewed vegetables, kitchen herbs, fruit, whole-grain products, vegetable oils with a high content of unsaturated sebacic or fatty acids, and milk products.

In spring, the experienced herb hunter thrusts dry grass aside, or lets himself be guided by the brownish-yellow stems of last year's growth, and there finds the bright green, fresh, new growth. Look for dandelions, yarrow, wild strawberries, stinging nettles, and plantain at this time of year.

The farther along into spring, the richer in content becomes the list of herb-foods—the dead nettle, St. John's-wort and ground ivy.

As autumn approaches, the leaves of the herbs get tougher and tougher. It is then advisable to gather only young shoots, if there are enough of them. Most effective are medicinal plants growing on untreated forest soil and not in chemically fertilized ground, or areas treated with chemical insecticides. From this you can see that you have to take a careful look at the place where you gather herbs and never pick them right at the edge of a field, in open country, nor on pastures or cultivated land. The person who has his own garden, which has not been treated with chemicals, is well off. Let your "weeds" remain standing and take for your daily needs only what you require—the "weed" ranks with the most valuable plants growing in the entire garden.

Other herbs can also be eaten fresh, but are not to be found everywhere, or only in particular seasons, as, for instance, sweet woodruff and wild thyme. Certain other plants are quite bitter and therefore not to everybody's taste, such as watercress and celandine.

When preparing herbs, the first thing to do is wash them, best with running water. Fresh herbs are more valuable in the preparation of teas than are dried herbs. This applies not only to the above-named medicinal plants, but also to other plants that bloom in the earliest part of the spring—colt's foot and chamomile.

DRYING

It is easy to lay aside a small supply of dried herbs for the winter. However, to dry and store up herbs in large quantities requires a great deal of specialized knowledge, which even goes so far as to include close observation of the phases of the moon, if a plant is to retain its full effectiveness.

For home use, only plants gathered in dry weather should be dried—neither rain-wet plants nor those wet with dew are suitable for long periods of storage. The strength of plants decreases as the time of day wears on—so gather them in the morning.

Only young leaves should be gathered, only blossoms that have just opened.

The drying that is absolutely necessary for storage of herbs is best done in a spot that is shady and exposed to the air—and the air must be dry. During extended periods of wet weather, farmers used to hang their herb harvest near the fireplace, but in such a way that the heat was not too close to the plants.

THE HERBARIUM

If you wish to establish a herbarium, you must keep in mind the same rule that holds good for gathering herbs for drying—gather only in dry, sunny weather. The pigment of the blossoms can be kept especially well if the plants are gathered in glaring sunshine and immediately pressed between sheets of blotting paper.

A few aids should be carried along when gathering herbs: two pieces of heavy cardboard measuring 30 × 35 cm (about 12 × 14 inches), between which you place sheets of blotting paper; some string for tying up the cardboards, a pocket knife; a garden trowel and, possibly, a net or cane for pulling water plants in to shore or for bringing tree branches down within reach.

Once a plant has been found, its identity is best checked with this guide book. Next, dig the plant out of the ground. Cut thick roots in half with the pocket knife. Heavy stems, too, can be handled the same way. Following this, carefully spread the plant out on blotting paper. If too many blossoms or leaves are present, so that they lie on top of each other, some of them may be removed. Plants that will not stay flat should be left to wither for a while and then they will be more tractable. Once the plant is laid out the way you want it, lay on one or more sheets of blotting paper, press the plant well, and then place the blotting-paper sandwich between the heavy cardboards and tie it securely with the string. Follow the same procedure with all plants collected. When you get home, place the cardboard packets under weights. Every day, change the position of the plants, exchanging the blotting paper that has meanwhile gotten damp, for dry sheets of the same.

After the plants are pressed (they are dry when they no longer feel cool) stick them down on paper. Use transparent tape, taping the plant down in several places. For the sake of security, mucilage can also be used in addition on small plant parts—for example, tender flower petals.

Next carefully label or caption the sheets of paper with plants attached. Identify by the Latin and the popular names, the place of discovery, the time of collection.

Spray lightly with an insecticide, so that the sheets do not fall victim to fungus and vermin.

Next cover the sheets with cellophane (or clear plastic) so that the plants will not suffer damage every time they are looked at. For a safe place to keep them, the best thing is a cardboard box, or thick portfolio.

HERB TEAS

A person in good health, making regular use of herb teas, must always take very small quantities, smaller than would be necessary to cure an illness. The mixing instructions in this book refer to dried herbs—fresh ones require greater quantities. The recommended mixture should never be increased and taken under the assumption that it will achieve a faster and more effective result.

If you want a quick result as, for example, in abdominal pains or a stomach disorder, it is advisable to take a small sip every 10 to 15 minutes and mix it well in your mouth with saliva before swallowing. Salivating is natural when eating and *drinking*. Therefore, do not bolt your food or gulp beverages down. The purpose of saliva is not merely to moisten the food in the stomach—it also contains enzymes which assimilate the food and make it available to the body's needs. Digestion begins in the mouth. This part of the digestive procedure cannot be made up for somewhere else in the body. If pressed for time, eat and drink less and devote yourself to better chewing.

Should a more acute condition be encountered, constipation, for instance, a cup of the appropriate herb tea will be enough.

In most cases, drinking a cup of herb tea three times daily and, of course, on an empty stomach, is effective when drunk at the latest a half-hour before lunch and a half-hour before dinner. Only a tea that has an especially stimulating effect on the gastric juices in the stomach should be administered a quarter-hour before a meal. Other teas thin the gastric juices when taken so shortly before mealtime, and thus create a stomach condition that is not receptive to the ingestion of food.

How long should such a course of herb-tea treatment last? When the illness in question has completely disappeared, you should continue to drink the tea for the same length of time that the illness itself was in effect, the time being reckoned from the day that the course of herb-tea treatment was begun.

Sugar should be entirely avoided during the herb-tea treatment and under no conditions should it be added to the tea. The body needs sugar, but only as a natural component of foods. In chemically isolated form, sugar causes a disturbance of the Vitamin-B balance. Such upsets cause others, primarily digestive difficulties. Teas, which are supposed to strengthen such digestive organs as the stomach, the liver, the gall bladder, or the intestine, are best enjoyed without any addition at all. On the other hand, teas taken for coughing can be improved with honey. However, not more than one teaspoonful of honey per day should be taken.

In the preparation of herb teas, it is important that the active ingredients not be destroyed, driven off or changed. The recommended quantities in this book apply to one cup of water. In general, if no instructions are given, consider the measure to be a level tablespoonful of the herb in question in a cup of water. A smaller quantity of herbs should be taken on days of good health; too much is, in any case, to be avoided.

You can make a cold infusion as well as a hot one. To do this, pour cold water over the herbs and allow to stand for about 12 hours. Strain the resulting herb beverage and warm it slightly for use.

A hot infusion can be obtained by pouring boiling water over the herbs. Stir and let stand about 5 minutes before straining. The tea is drunk when its temperature has dropped to about body temperature (98.6°F = 37°C).

A tea is called a "decoction" when the herbs are put into cold water, which is then brought to a boil and kept at the boiling point for 5 minutes over moderate heat. It is then strained and drunk at body temperature.

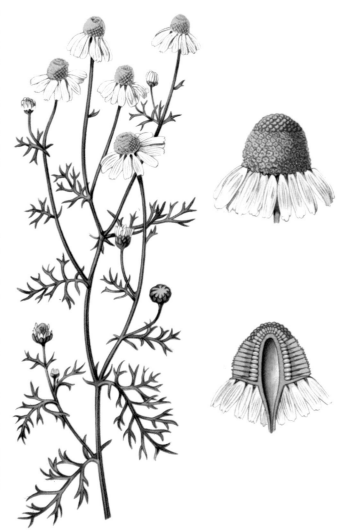

Wild Chamomile

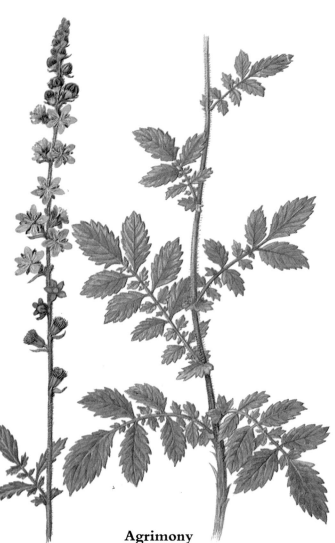

Agrimony

AGRIMONY

SCIENTIFIC NAME: *Agrimonia eupatoria*.

OTHER POPULAR NAMES: Common agrimony, liverwort, sticklewort, cockleburr.

FAMILY: Rosaceae—Rose Family.

RANGE: Along fences, hedges, roadsides, and on slopes, agrimony shoots up its mullein-like, golden flower spike. This perennial plant is native to Europe, but is now found in Canada and the United States, along roadsides and in fields and woods, flowering in July or August.

DESCRIPTION: From a short root-stock, the plant rises vertically to a height of up to 80 cm (32 inches). The grey-green, pinnate leaves give off a light, pleasant scent when rubbed between the fingers. A long-lasting dense flower spike develops, with many small golden blossoms surrounded by thorny calyxes.

ELEMENTS CONTAINED: Tannin, a bitter principle (an ingredient imparting a characteristic quality), some essential oil, in the ashes rather a lot of silicic acid, nicotic (nicotinic) acid amide (a complex of nicotinamide), which is the vitamin whose deficiency causes pellagra.

MEDICINAL USE: The plant—*Herba Agrimoniae*.

In classical antiquity, this plant was used internally for liver and gall-bladder troubles. Today agrimony is used externally in the treatment of wounds and ulcers. It is also valued in cases of diarrhea and digestive disturbance. Skin troubles, too, are beneficially influenced, and it has a stimulating effect on the kidneys and the elimination of uric acid.

CULINARY USE: None.

ANGELICA

SCIENTIFIC NAME: *Angelica archangelica.*
OTHER POPULAR NAMES: Garden angelica, Holy Ghost.
FAMILY: Umbelliferae—Parsley or Carrot Family.
RANGE: There are two varieties of *Angelica archangelica.* The sub-species *eu-archangelica* occurs in the mountain country of northern lands, such as Iceland, Greenland and Scandinavia; the second subspecies, *littoralis,* is a beach plant of Greenland, Iceland, Scandinavia, the Russian Baltic seacoast and Siberia. This plant was grown in European convent and monastery gardens during the Middle Ages.

The American angelica is *Angelica atropurpurea* which grows 1.2–1.8 metres (4–6 feet) high and has begonia-like leaves. It is found in swamps from Newfoundland to Delaware and Minnesota. Umbels as large as 10 inches (25 cm) across.

DESCRIPTION: In the first year of its growth and into the autumn, angelica is a stemless plant with triply pinnate leaves (triply divided into leaflets) almost a metre (about 40 inches) long growing from the strongly developed root. The following summer, however, the plant shoots upward, sending up a hollow, thick stalk with pinnate leaves sprouting from bulbous leaf sheaths, and branches ending in greenish-yellow flattened flower clusters called umbels.

ELEMENTS CONTAINED: Cane sugar, some starch, hydrocarotin, angelic acid, valeric acid, malic acid, resin, tannin, pectin, wax, a bitter principle, and up to 1 per cent essential oil.

MEDICINAL PARTS: The leaves—*Foliae Angelicae*; the root—*Radix Angelicae.* All parts of the plant promote perspiration and urination and stimulate the appetite and nerves. Angelica has been used in folk medicine, except for plague, as an expectorant in cases of obstruction by mucus, against constipation caused by hemorrhoids and to treat jaundice, to calm the heart and in cases of insomnia. As a preventative, the tea is drunk when there is danger of catching cold. To make tea, scald by pouring 1 cup of boiling water over 1–2 grams (15.4–30.8 grains avdp) of the leaves, 2–4 grams (1–2 level teaspoonfuls) of the root, or 1–2 grams (15.4–30.8 grains avdp) of the seeds. The root and seeds may be briefly boiled.

CULINARY USE: The stems can be jellied or candied, cooked with rhubarb, blanched like celery, boiled, or cooked with sugar, like fruit. The roots can also be boiled or preserved. The leaves can

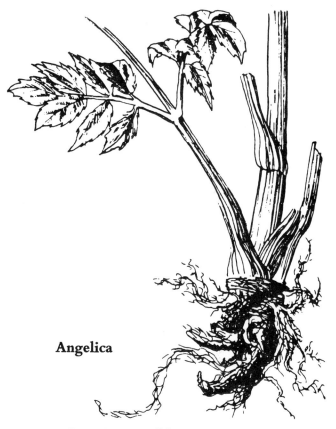

Angelica

(Also see illustration, page 122)

be candied or served with fish. In Lapland, angelica has been chewed and smoked like tobacco. The American Indians smoked it straight, or mixed it with tobacco. The seeds and an oil from the stem are used in making Benedictine, Chartreuse, vermouth and other alcoholic drinks, as well as in creams and custards. The roots are used in making Chartreuse.

ANISE

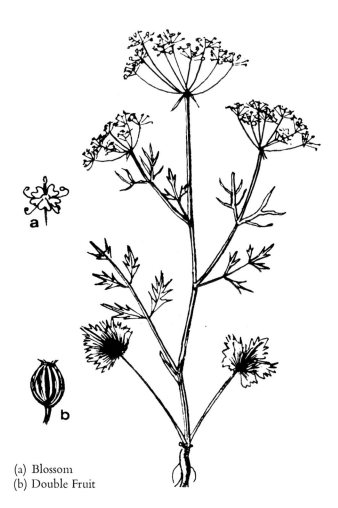

(a) Blossom
(b) Double Fruit

Anise

SCIENTIFIC NAME: *Pimpinella anisum.*

OTHER POPULAR NAMES: Aniseed, sweet cumin.

FAMILY: Umbelliferae—Parsley or Carrot Family.

RANGE: Native to the Mediterranean region, this plant has been cultivated from ancient times and today is grown mainly in Spain and Russia. It likes dry climatic conditions.

DESCRIPTION: In the first year, a rosette of leaves first grows out of the spindle-shaped root, as usual among the Umbelliferae. The following year, the plant sends up a round, furrowed stem whose lower leaves are almost undivided, while the upper ones are progressively more deeply cut with progressively smaller pinnae. The stalk branches and at the end of each is a fluffy, white umbel.

ELEMENTS CONTAINED: The fruits contain 2–3 per cent essential oil, along with protein, fat, and sugar.

MEDICINAL USE: Fruit—*Fructus Anisi;* oil—*Oleum Anisi.* Anise has a strongly antispasmodic effect and is carminative, that is, it strongly counters flatulency; it is an expectorant; it soothes pain and mitigates coughing. It is used for loss of appetite, difficulty of digestion, mucus obstruction in coughs and whooping cough, and stomach and intestinal troubles. A decoction of 2–4 grams (30.8–61.6 grains avdp—$\frac{3}{4}$–$1\frac{1}{2}$ teaspoons) of the seeds in 1 cup of water promotes milk secretion. It is also used to spice medicines, such as paregoric.

CULINARY USE: Anise has an aromatic, sweetish taste and makes pastry and bread more easily digestible. The dried dehiscent fruit (schizocarp) of the anise plant is used for making bread, pastries, and cookies; to season vegetables and salads; and in milk, desserts, plum jam, brandy and cordials. Use up ground anise quickly, since its strength deteriorates rapidly.

ARNICA

SCIENTIFIC NAME: *Arnica montana.*

OTHER POPULAR NAMES: Leopard's bane, fall dandelion, mountain tobacco, mountain arnica.

FAMILY: Compositae—Composite Family.

RANGE: Almost everywhere in Europe in damp, peaty meadows, forest clearings, and mountain meadows of the Alps, up to an altitude of 2,000 m (about 6,500 feet). It is also found in Canada and the northern United States.

DESCRIPTION: Near the ground is a rosette of a few plantain-like, paired leaves, each with 5–7 veins, from whose midst a slender stem rises, ending in a flower bud. The stem often has a pair of tiny leaves, from the axes of which sprout two other stems, complete with flower buds. When the sun reaches its highest annual position in the sky, the composite yellow flower head comes into bloom, the disc flowers in the middle, wreathed around with shining ray flowers. After blooming is over, the wind sows the silvery seed around. At this time, the root-stock develops horizontal rootlets that produce buds at their ends. Next spring, these will unfold into new leaf rosettes and the cycle of growth will begin again.

ELEMENTS CONTAINED: Tannic acid is found in all parts of the plant. In the blossoms is flavone (a yellow plant pigment), a carotin-like pigment (arnicerin), choline, an essential oil that counters inflammation, silicic acid, inulin and arnica. The root contains a skin-irritating, volatile oil, gummy substances, wax, inulin and arnicin. The plant itself contains the same elements but is hardly ever used.

MEDICINAL USE: Blossoms—*Flores Arnicae*; root—*Radix Arnicae*; whole plant—*Herba Arnicae*.

The designation "Radix" in this case may certainly be used but is misleading, for the entire root-stock is used. It should more correctly be named *Rhizoma Arnicae*.

Arnica is used externally in the form of a tincture but only in an aqueous dilution (1:2 to 1:6). It is effective in cases of sprains and dislocations, bruises and contusions (but not safe if skin is broken as tincture is poisonous), extravasation (internal or external bleeding), and excoriations (abrasions of the skin), for alleviating pain, promoting resorption (assimilation of material into the blood or lymph systems) and countering inflammation.

Rubbing in thinned arnica tincture has a beneficial effect on gout, rheumatism, and stiffness. Moreover, it strengthens and invigorates the nerves.

Arnica is also used internally as a tincture in a dilution of 20 drops of arnica tincture to a fourth of a litre (about $8\frac{1}{2}$ oz) of water. Take a sip of this solution every two hours. Too frequent or stronger doses can cause poisoning, probably owing to the arnica. Because of this, internal use should be supervised by a physician. The internal doses amplify the effect of external applications and have a lasting effect on the nerves, heart and blood circulation. Naturopathic physicians give injections of arnica.

CULINARY USE: None.

(See illustration, page 2)

Artemisia

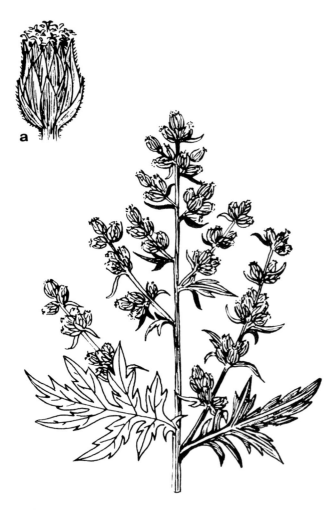

SCIENTIFIC NAME: *Artemisia vulgaris, A. ludoviciana* (U.S.).

POPULAR NAMES: Mugwort, wormwood, common artemisia, sagebrush (U.S.).

FAMILY: Compositae—Composite Family.

RANGE: Artemisia is found in all parts of Europe, in hedges, along fences and walls, in uncultivated places, fallow fields, on slopes and on the banks of streams. It is native also to Asia and naturalized in eastern North America.

DESCRIPTION: The plant grows to a height of about 60 cm (24 inches) from a thin, brown root which is white inside. The plant is bushy and multi-branched, with numerous leaves, green on top and white and felt-like on the underside. Ordinary artemisia has erect, composite blossoms.

ELEMENTS CONTAINED: A bitter principle, essential oil, tannic acid.

MEDICINAL USE: The plant—*Herba Artemisiae*; the root—*Radix Artemisiae*.

To counter epilepsy, give 1–2 grams (15.4–30.8 grains avdp) in a glass of water as an infusion (pouring boiling water upon) or a light decoction (boiled briefly); or in powder form, 1 teaspoonful daily, mixed into a beverage. Artemisia is also effective in counterbalancing disorders of the menstrual period, if it is taken 3–8 days before the commencement of the period. Artemisia has a neutralizing effect on fatty foods, acts as a sedative and a diuretic. As a tea (1 teaspoonful of artemisia boiled in 1 cup of water), it is effective as a sedative and a sudorific (promoter of perspiration).

CULINARY USE: This herb is also esteemed as a culinary seasoning, especially used with roast goose.

Artemisia is pleasantly spicy with a somewhat bitter tang. Use the fresh or dried buds (entire panicles). A bunch of fresh artemisia can be cooked with meat, or the dried herb or a powder form of it can be added.

It is especially suitable for fat meat dishes: roast pork, goose or duck; roast wild boar; eel, pan gravy, pickles, sauerbraten (beef soaked in vinegar and cooked in a stew pan). Green artemisia is used in salads.

(a) Flower head (= floret)

Artemisia

Autumn Crocus

SCIENTIFIC NAME: *Colchicum autumnale.*

OTHER POPULAR NAMES: Meadow saffron, wild saffron, colchicum, meadow crocus.

FAMILY: Liliaceae—Lily Family.

RANGE: In Europe, in the Mediterranean region, and in the Orient, the autumn crocus grows everywhere, spread out over the meadows singly and in groups. It has been naturalized in some areas of the United States.

DESCRIPTION: The autumn crocus is not a true crocus—true crocuses belong to the Iris Family. In comparison with other plants, the autumn crocus leads a life diametrically opposed to the rhythm of the year. From September to October, everywhere on the meadows the pale violet blossoms announce the advent of winter. These blossoms rise directly out of the bulb, without the transitional phase of leaves. The process of the flower remains imbedded in the root since the 3-part fruiting arrangement lies hidden deep in a lateral groove of the root. The long-tubed, funnel-shaped perigonium (a type of petal formation) is divided at the top into 6 crown-points and bears in its throat 6 stamens grown together. The pollen, which germinates from the stigma upon pollination, requires many weeks before it turns into egg-cells in the seed-bud.

Fructification does not occur until Christmas. Sheltered from frost in the bulb under the earth, the seed develops during the winter. In the spring, when other plants are blooming, the fruit-bearing stem with tulip-like leaves climbs upward toward the light, so that, in the following summer, the 3-part fruit capsules with their ridged seeds can mature.

ELEMENTS CONTAINED: The principal constituent develops in all parts of the plant, but especially in the seeds. This is colchicine, the strongest mitotic poison we know of. Treatment of plant seeds with colchicine leads to erratic mutations.

MEDICINAL USE: The seeds—*Semen Colchici.*

On account of the plant's poisonous character, it should be taken only on prescription from a physician. The medieval Swedish philosopher, Albertus Magnus, recommended it for gout. In cases of over-acidity of the organism and all the consequences thereof, such as gout and rheumatism, treatment with colchicum is applied. However, it also has a beneficial effect on

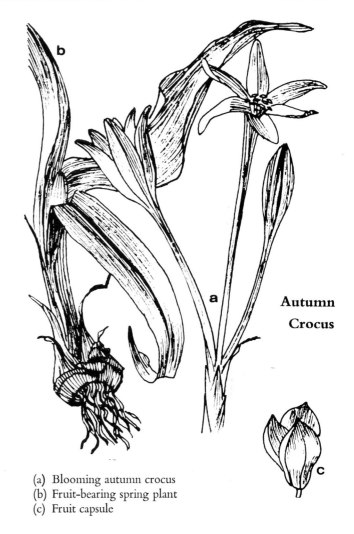

Autumn Crocus

(a) Blooming autumn crocus
(b) Fruit-bearing spring plant
(c) Fruit capsule

European (or summer) cholera, dropsy, and tumor of the thyroid gland. In former times, people used the seeds to drive away lice.

CULINARY USE: None. Poisonous.

Avens

AVENS

SCIENTIFIC NAME: *Geum urbanum.*

OTHER POPULAR NAMES: Wood avens, common avens, herb bennet, bennet, yellow avens, blessed herb, star of the earth.

FAMILY: Rosaceae—Rose Family.

RANGE: In the north temperate zone, this plant thrives along walls and fences, on damp rubbish and stone heaps, and in woods, hedges, and shady places.

DESCRIPTION: The finger-thick, pinkish root-stock emits a scent reminiscent of cloves. It develops a rosette of regular, roundish, pinnate leaves which, as they approach the top of the stem, become simpler, at first still three-lobed, but next to the golden-yellow, early-summer blossoms, they are only spiniform (like spines).

ELEMENTS CONTAINED: A bitter principle, tannin, eugenol (source of the spicy, clove-like smell), essential oil, resin, starch, gum and flavone.

MEDICINAL USE: The root—*Radix Caryophillatae.*

Avens tea is used externally. Make it from 1–3 grams (15.4–46.2 grains avdp) of the root, scalded with 1 cup of boiling water, or briefly boiled. Use as a gargle for inflammation of the mouth and throat, for it is hemostatic (blood-stanching), an anodyne (pain-reducing), and a germicidal agent. The internal effect of avens restricts the development of viruses. This characteristic and the tannin are certainly a substantial aid in cases of diarrhea and colic. At work here, too, is its nerve-strengthening influence, which operates in the region of the stomach and intestines. In obstructions and disturbances of secretions of the liver and the gall bladder, avens has proved itself. The tea used to be given as a strengthening agent in conditions of exhaustion and after severe illness.

CULINARY USE: Whole and ground, avens has the spicy scent of carnation; a sharp, fiery taste. Use dried. Boil the whole plant with rest of ingredients, remove after cooking is done, or sprinkle avens powder sparingly while cooking.

Used in Christmas cakes, in mulled claret, with game and mutton, and in soups, sauces, marinades, cabbage dishes (sauerkraut), preserves, soufflés, drinks, and as seasoning for canning. Keep in tightly closed container. Has a stomachic effect.

LEMON BALM

SCIENTIFIC NAME: *Melissa officinalis*.

POPULAR NAMES: Bee balm, balm, balm mint, melissa, garden-balm, sweet-balm.

FAMILY: Labiatae—Mint Family.

RANGE: The bee and this plant have been given the same name in Greek (melissa), because bees prefer the nectar of lemon balm. In the Orient, where the plant originated, it has often been cultivated over wide areas as food for bees. The Arabs brought it to Spain and the Benedictine monks carried it into Germany, where it was cultivated in monastery and pharmaceutical gardens. Today, lemon balm is cultivated widely throughout the world. In the eastern United States, it has become naturalized.

DESCRIPTION: The perennial root with many short runners sends forth a branched, square stem that is slightly hairy. The leaves are set in opposed pairs, rising one above the other. From the top-most leaf axes a few white blossoms emerge, rich in nectar.

ELEMENTS CONTAINED: 0.25–1 per cent essential oil, containing citral (citron + aldehyde) and citronella (a terpene aldehyde) which give it its lemon-like scent.

MEDICINAL USE: Leaves—*Folia Melissae*; plant—*Herba Melissae*.

Lemon balm has a general effect on the digestive tract. Its specific effect is stimulating, antispasmodic, sedative, anti-flatulent and relieves both vomiting and nausea. Also, palpitation of the heart, heart neuroses, sleeplessness, hysteria, menstrual disturbances, and sexually irritating conditions are beneficially influenced. Lemon-balm tea is prepared by taking 2–4 grams (30.8–61.6 grains avdp) of the leaves or the entire plant and scalding them with 1 cup of boiling water. (Never allow the tea to boil.)

CULINARY USE: Formerly, sprigs of lemon balm, freshly picked, were put into drinks in warm weather. In France a liqueur is made from lemon balm—*eau de mélisse*, or melissa cordial.

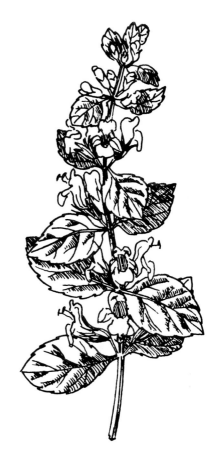

Lemon Balm

SWEET BASIL

SCIENTIFIC NAME: *Ocimum basilicum*.

OTHER POPULAR NAMES: Common basil, St. Josephwort.

FAMILY: Labiatae—Mint Family.

RANGE: This plant, native to India was known to the ancient Egyptians, for wreaths of basil have been found in the burial chambers of the pyramids. The Greeks esteemed basil as both a medicinal and a food-spicing plant. It is cultivated in all parts of Europe today, as well as in tropical Asia, the Americas, Africa and the Pacific Islands.

DESCRIPTION: This annual herb is multi-branched and bushy and grows to a height of about 40 cm (16 inches). It has broad, somewhat fleshy leaves. The leaf shoots end in whorls of white flowers.

ELEMENTS CONTAINED: The principal component is an essential oil.

MEDICINAL USE: The entire plant—*Herba Basilici*. Basil has been long known as a remedy for soothing pain, for promoting perspiration (sudorific), and it has a sedative effect. It is used for stomach cramps, bladder and kidney troubles, and to promote the production of mother's milk, as well as in cases of nervous debility (neurasthenia).

CULINARY USES: Basil is aromatic, cool, sweetish and spicy, with a somewhat hot after-taste. If used dried, keep well sealed; if fresh, chop the leaves fine. Basil is used in salads, gravies, un-cooked (vegetarian) food, dishes made from curds; pork, mutton and veal dishes; fish and highly seasoned cocktails. It is the classic seasoning for tomato dishes.

Sweet Basil

BEARBERRY

SCIENTIFIC NAME: *Arbutus uva-ursi* (*Arctostaphylos uva-ursi*).

OTHER POPULAR NAMES: Kinnikinnik (American Indian name), uva-ursi, upland cranberry, arberry, common bearberry.

FAMILY: Ericaceae—Heath Family.

RANGE: Throughout central Europe, northern Asia and North America in coniferous forests and on heaths. Bearberry is found among water-soaked, succulent cushions of pale-green turf moss as well as on stretches of sandy soil. It has leathery, evergreen, fragile oval leaves clinging to many-branched limbs. The pitcher-shaped blossoms, edged with white and red, are 5-pointed and terminal (situated at the tip). In early summer, they change into the purplish-red, berry-like fruits.

ELEMENTS CONTAINED: Arbutin, methylarbutin, a bitter principle, ursolic acid, tannic acid, gallic acid, some essential oil and resin.

MEDICINAL USE: Leaves—*Folia Uvae Ursi*.

Bearberry-leaf tea (2–5 grams in a cup of boiling water) (30.8–77 grains avdp) is a first-rate remedy for catarrh of the bladder, kidney trouble such as gravel in the kidneys, and kidney stones. It also has a salutary effect on bed-wetting (enuresis). Combined with tobacco for smoking, it was used as a headache cure by the Chippewa Indians.

CULINARY USE: None. The berries were part of the diet of eastern American Indians; bears also like them. The Indians and the early settlers smoked the dried leaves, sometimes mixed with other herbs or tobacco.

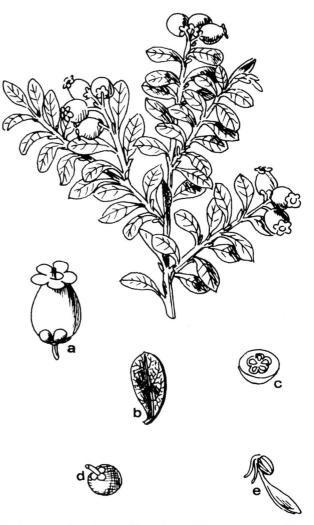

(a) Blossom enlarged   (b) Leaf   (c) Cross-section of fruit
(d) Fruit   (e) Stamen

Bearberry

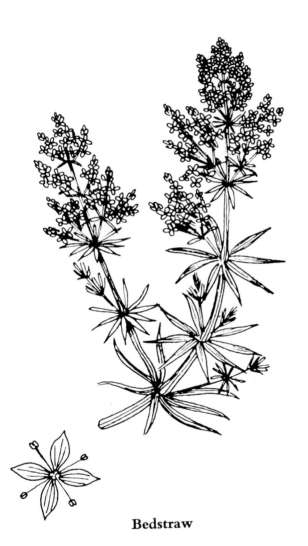

Bedstraw

BEDSTRAW

SCIENTIFIC NAME: *Galium aparine* or any species of this genus.

OTHER POPULAR NAMES: Cleavers, goose grass, catch weed, clivers, hariff, scratch weed, cleaverwort, Our Lady's bedstraw.

FAMILY: Rubiaceae—Madder Family.

RANGE: Bedstraw, of which there are many species, grows everywhere along fences, roadsides and field borders. Common to Europe and the United States, it grows in cultivated grounds, moist thickets, and along banks of rivers.

DESCRIPTION: This plant climbs man-high from leaf-whorl to leaf-whorl and holds itself fast to fences and bushes with its backward-growing bristles. The small, whitish-green blossoms, compressed into cymes, are only weakly developed. The spherical little fruits stick like burrs to clothing, since they are thickly set with tiny hooks.

The name, Our Lady's bedstraw, is applied more often to the non-sticking species. In the Middle Ages, it was believed that the Virgin Mary placed this plant in the manger when she laid the Christ Child down to sleep. Bedstraw species also contain a rennet enzyme (a saponin) that causes milk to curdle. Greek shepherds made a kind of sieve out of bedstraw and poured milk through it to promote its curdling.

ELEMENTS CONTAINED: Saponins, rubichloric acid, silicic acid, citric acid, tannic acid, red dyestuff.

MEDICINAL USE: The plant—*Herba Galii aparinis*.

The saponin makes bedstraw a diuretic (inducing the flow of urine) and a phlegm-raising agent. For this reason, it is given for kidney complaints and dropsy, as well as in cases of pleurisy, chronic skin eruptions, and liver troubles. For tea, 2–4 grams (30.8–61.6 grains avdp) of the dried plant are scalded with 1 cup of boiling water, never boiled.

CULINARY USE: Used to curdle milk.

Bindweed

SCIENTIFIC NAMES: *Convolvulus arvensis* (field-bindweed); *Convolvulus sepium* (fence-bindweed).

OTHER POPULAR NAMES: Small bindweed, field-bindweed, lesser bindweed *(C. arvensis)*, Rutland Beauty, great bindweed, convolvulus, calystegia, larger bindweed, greater bindweed, bearbind *(C. sepium)*.

FAMILY: Convolvulaceae—Morning-Glory Family.

RANGE: Bindweed is encountered throughout central Europe along roadsides, fences, in grain fields, along hedges and the banks of streams. *C. arvensis* is naturalized in America, sometimes used decoratively in hanging baskets, etc. *C. sepium* is found in Europe, Asia, and North America.

DESCRIPTION: True to its name, bindweed winds itself in tight spirals around stalks of grain, fence posts, bushes and trees, and beautifies many a rubbish dump or rail fence with its white to pale-pink funnel-shaped blossoms, which, after blooming, roll up spirally. The pink coloration (which indicates the presence of iron in the soil) is offset by 5 snow-white stripes from the yellowish flower base to the edge. In bad weather, the flower closes its calyx which, in the sunshine, lures insects with its delicate, pleasant aroma to the orange-tinted ovaries, which are so guarded by the 5 stamens that the invader must take pollen away with it, if it wishes to reach the sweet nectar.

ELEMENTS CONTAINED: Resin and the glycoside jalapin.

MEDICINAL USE: The plant—*Herba Convolvuli*; root and plant—*Herba et Radix Convolvuli*.

Bindweed used to be a prized purgative. The tea is made from 2–4 grams (30.8–61.6 grains avdp) of the plant with flowers after scalding with 1 cup of boiling water; or, the plant with the root is briefly boiled in 1 cup of water. It acts as a purgative and cholagogic (induces a flow of bile), without having the strong irritating effect on the bowels of such herbal remedies as jalap *(Exogonium purga)* or senna leaves *(Folia sennae)*. The use of these latter species in cases of catarrh (inflammation) of the intestinal mucous membrane, and mucous discharge is not harmless—in case of a sensitive intestine, they can lead to blockage of the colon.

CULINARY USE: None.

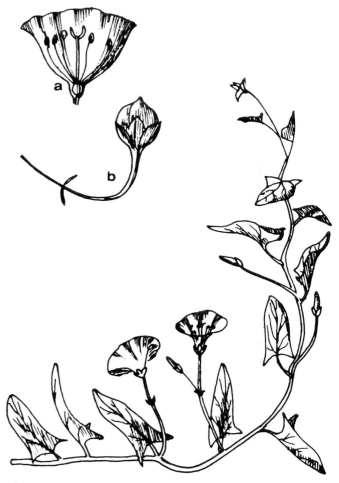

(a) Cross-section of a flower
(b) Fruit

Bindweed

BIRTHWORT

SCIENTIFIC NAME: *Aristolochia clematitis.*

OTHER POPULAR NAME: Upright birthwort.

FAMILY: Aristolochiaceae—Birthwort Family.

RANGE: Birthwort was valued by the ancient Greeks and Romans as a medicinal plant. It is native to the warm lands around the Mediterranean Sea. From there, it came to northern Europe rather early, along with the cultivation of grapes, and adapted itself to the climate. Today, it grows wild along European hedges and fences, and is naturalized in the eastern United States.

DESCRIPTION: The metre-high (40-inch-high) climbing (with tendrils) shrub has heart-shaped, stemmed leaves and distinctive, yellow blossoms. Behind a long perigonium-tube with downward-directed hairs, a pistil and 6 stamens lie in a thickened part, so grown together that pollen cannot succeed in reaching the stigma. At this point, small flies take over as intermediaries. With the pollen of other plants of the same species, they fly down into the tube and become captives of the flower, for the downward-directed hairs will not let them out again. The insects fly excitedly about until they have wiped off their pollen on the 6-lobed stigma. Not until then do the hairs flatten out and permit the captives to escape.

ELEMENTS CONTAINED: The most active constituent is aristolochiaceous acid.

MEDICINAL USE: The plant—*Herba Aristolochiae*; the root—*Radix Aristolochiae longae.*

Everywhere throughout the world the birthwort and its various relatives have enjoyed the highest reputation as medicinal plants. The snake charmers of India and North Africa believe that a drop of the juice of the birthwort will kill any snake, and that people who rub themselves with the juice make themselves immune to snakebite. As a blood-purifying agent, birthwort has its place in folk medicine. It was formerly used against wounds, suppuration and bloody discharge following birth, which is what its name means (*aristos* = best; *locheia* = birth).

Modern science has now discovered how the effect of this medicinal plant comes about. Aristolochiaceous acid strengthens the function of the leucocytes in resisting infection. In the first place, its effect is to increase their number markedly and, in the second place, to increase their power to kill germs. At the same

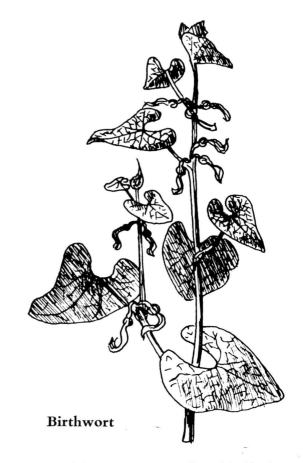

Birthwort

time, the natural, bacteria-restraining effect of the blood serum is activated. This biological process also assists the organism without burdening it.

Mix 2 tablespoonfuls of the plant or root and briefly boil them in $\frac{1}{2}$ litre (1 pint) of water. Wet poultices can be made from this decoction for badly healing wounds and ulcers. Since aristolochiaceous acid can now be isolated in pure form, it is also nowadays given internally, so as to assist in the healing of wounds that are difficult to reach from the outside.

CULINARY USE: None.

BORAGE

SCIENTIFIC NAME: *Borago officinalis.*

OTHER POPULAR NAMES: Burrage, common bugloss, bee-plant, bee bread, star flower, common borage.

FAMILY: Boraginaceae—Borage Family.

RANGE: Native to the Mediterranean region, borage is mostly found in gardens in northern Europe, and is widely naturalized elsewhere as a weed. In many cases, it is also found growing wild on refuse dumps and on damp soil rich in humus.

DESCRIPTION: This annual, coarsely haired plant unfolds its abundant foliage and gleaming blue flowers in summer, which in blossoming bend heavily toward the earth. The fast, vigorous growth responds to the earth's gravity, a fact that is visible in its general drooping appearance.

ELEMENTS CONTAINED: Traces of essential oil; mucilaginous matter, tannic acid, saponin, silicic acid, malic-acidulous lime, and potassium nitrate.

MEDICINAL USE: Borage leaves—*Folia Boraginis*; borage blossoms—*Flores Boraginis.*

The blossoms have a strengthening effect on the heart. The plant is employed in cases of mycodermitis, phlebitis, and congestion. It is best used raw, chopped into fine pieces and mixed in with a vegetable salad. To prepare a tea, take 1 teaspoonful of the dried herb and pour over it 1 cup of boiling water.

CULINARY USE: Has a strong, onion-like smell and a spicy, cucumber-like taste. When used fresh, the leaves and blossoms should be finely chopped. The dried herb should be ground or powdered and should be kept well sealed.

Borage can be added to cabbage-type vegetables, gravies, dishes of yogurt mixtures, and spiced punches. In some parts of France, the flowers are dipped in batter and fried to make fritters.

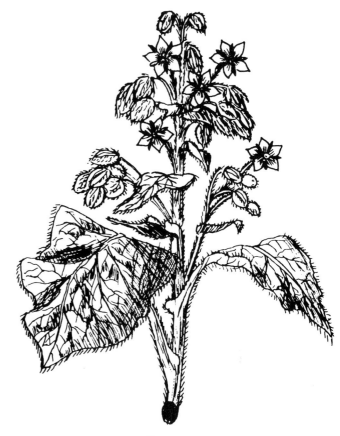

Borage

Buckbean

SCIENTIFIC NAME: *Menyanthes trifoliata.*

OTHER POPULAR NAMES: Bogbean, bog myrtle, water shamrock, marsh trefoil.

FAMILY: Gentianaceae—the Gentian Family. (Some authors separate it into the family Menyanthaceae—the Buckbean Family.)

RANGE: Buckbean is to be found throughout the entire northern hemisphere, wherever the ground is wet and marshy.

DESCRIPTION: From a long, creeping root-stock, the stem rises to a height of about 30 cm (12 inches). Long-stemmed, trifoliate leaves play around the stem, which is crowned by a pale reddish cluster of blossoms rising above the water. It ceases to flower by late summer.

ELEMENTS CONTAINED: Glycosidic bitter principle, fat oil, choline, phosphoric acid.

MEDICINAL USE: The leaves—*Folia Trifolii fibrini.*

Buckbean is used only internally. Scald 5 grams (77 grains avdp) by pouring over the leaf $\frac{1}{2}$ litre (about 17 oz) of boiling water and let it steep for $\frac{1}{2}$ hour before straining. The tea is given for digestive disturbances, as an appetite stimulator, and for liver troubles, $\frac{1}{2}$ hour before meals. It is also esteemed as a remedy for fever and migraine.

CULINARY USE: The large, starchy roots of the buckbean are said to be used in northern Scandinavia to make a nutritious flour.

Buckbean

GREAT BURDOCK

SCIENTIFIC NAME: *Arctium lappa (Lappa major, L. edulis).*
OTHER POPULAR NAMES: Bardana, clotburr, common burdock.
FAMILY: Compositae—Composite Family.
RANGE: Burdock is widespread throughout all parts of the world, growing as a trash plant along fences, roadsides, and on earth heaps.
DESCRIPTION: Burdock is commonly found in the vicinity of human dwellings. There the powerful root bores as much as half a metre (20 inches) downward into wet rubbish. Burdocks like an abundance of light, and with their large, heart-shaped ground leaves, they cover otherwise unsightly ground. The sturdy stem branches out into an abundantly leaved bush, from which climb corymbs (erect clusters) of violet blossoms. The latter are beloved by children on account of their hooklike crooked, involucral scales (burrs), by means of which the flower heads attach themselves to clothing and hair and are difficult to remove. In the same manner, the seeds are also spread abroad by animals in whose fur the burrs cling.
ELEMENTS CONTAINED: 40–50 per cent inulin, 5 per cent glucose, mucilage, essential oil, resin, tannin, 3–4 per cent mineral substances, 12 per cent raw protein, stigmasterol and sitosterol.
MEDICINAL USE: The root—*Radix Bardanae.*

As a powerful diaphoretic (sweat-inducing agent) and diuretic, burdock is used with greatest effect against gout, rheumatism and skin diseases. A tea is brewed from 3–5 grams (46.2–77 grains avdp) in 1 cup of boiling water, or boiled briefly.

Its external use as a hair-growing agent has been known from ancient times. Paracelsus, the Swiss physician of the 16th century, himself recommended burdock in this respect. As a blood-purifying agent, it is an ingredient of blood-purifying teas (species Lignorum).
CULINARY USE: Burdock is cultivated in Japan as a garden vegetable, for its edible leaf stalks, flower stalks and roots.

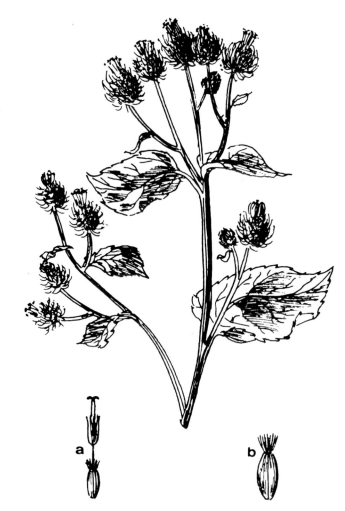

(a) Blossom
(b) Fruit

Great Burdock

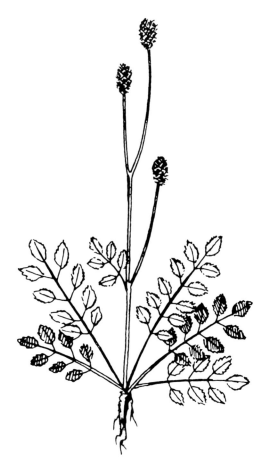

Burnet

BURNET

SCIENTIFIC NAME: *Sanguisorba officinalis.*

OTHER POPULAR NAMES: Greater burnet, great burnet, common burnet, garden burnet, Italian burnet, Italian pimpernel.

FAMILY: Rosaceae—Rose Family.

RANGE: This plant is found on rather wet meadows in central Europe, as far north as Norway, as well as in Asia; to some degree naturalized in North America.

DESCRIPTION: From a vigorous root-stock grows a rosette of simple, pinnate, unpaired leaves, out of the middle of which springs a bare, long stem. Walking through the meadows, we especially notice the brown flower heads projecting from the grass. The great burnet is not to be mistaken for its double, the lesser burnet *(Sanguisorba minor)*, which differs from the greater burnet in that its flower heads possess a reddish glimmer, derived from the projecting red stigmas (actually, the flowers are green and not brown).

ELEMENTS CONTAINED: Rich in tannin, saponin.

MEDICINAL USE: The plant—*Herba Sanguisorbae.*

Used for stanching internal bleeding, bleeding of the lungs, stomach and intestines, and bleeding of non-malignant tumors and hemorrhoids.

CULINARY USE: The young leaves can be added to salads. In the United States, the Pennsylvania Dutch (i.e. Germans) steeped burnet leaves in tankards to make a drink called "cool cup."

Sanguisorba minor is also called Italian pimpernel because, on account of its cucumber-like taste, it is added to wine in Italy to improve its aroma. It is considered a garden herb for seasoning sauces and soups.

Burnet Saxifrage

SCIENTIFIC NAME: *Pimpinella saxifraga.*
OTHER POPULAR NAME: Common pimpinel (obs. pimpernel).
FAMILY: Umbelliferae—Parsley or Carrot Family.
RANGE: Throughout central Europe, *Pimpinella saxifraga* occurs on dry meadows, pastures and hills.

Burnet saxifrage must not be confused with the lesser burnet, *Sanguisorba minor*, which is popular as a kitchen herb and has leaves that are quite similar to *Pimpinella saxifraga* and its large variety, *Pimpinella major*.

ELEMENTS CONTAINED: Tannin, sugar, albumen, essential oil, gum, starch, saponin, benzoic acid, a bitter principle, pimpinellin.
MEDICINAL USE: The root—*Radix Pimpinellae.*

Burnet saxifrage causes secretion of mucus and stimulates skin and kidneys. It was formerly employed as a remedy for kidney and bladder stones. Even a beneficial effect on the liver has been ascribed to it. Folk medicine also used it in cases of dropsy and tuberculosis. The root of the burnet saxifrage is given to counter hoarseness—1–3 grams (15.4–46.2 grains avdp) in 1 cup water, as a light decoction.
CULINARY USE: None.

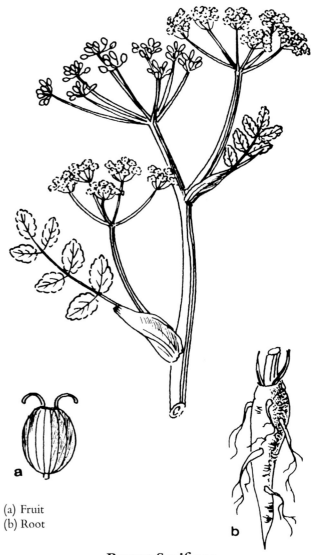

(a) Fruit
(b) Root

Burnet Saxifrage

CARAWAY

SCIENTIFIC NAME: *Carum carvi.*

OTHER POPULAR NAME: Common caraway.

FAMILY: Umbelliferae—Parsley or Carrot Family.

RANGE: Caraway grows wild in Europe from the Alps as far north as Norway and also is found in northern and central Asia and has been naturalized in parts of North America. It thrives on wet meadows, field borders, alluvial land and slopes. In many regions, it is also cultivated.

DESCRIPTION: In the first year of its growth, caraway sends up an abundant foliage of carrot-like leaves and also develops a fleshy root that looks very much like a carrot. In the second year, the stalks shoot up quickly and their umbels are soon blooming when spring withdraws. The umbels and umbellets (small umbels composing an umbel) have no involucral leaflets (resembling a calyx) and it is characteristic of the white-blooming umbel that it develops higher umbellets at the edge than in the middle.

ELEMENTS CONTAINED: 3–7 per cent essential oil, waxes, resin. The ashes yield a great deal of silicic acid and iron oxide, as well as magnesium oxide.

MEDICINAL USE: The fruit—*Fructus Carvi*; oil—*Oleum Carvi.*

Caraway has a powerful effect on the stomach and intestines and stimulates the digestive glands. Metabolism is enlivened. Flatulence is expelled; moreover, stomach and uterine cramps are obviated. A decoction of 4–5 grams (2–$2\frac{1}{2}$ teaspoonfuls or 61.6–77 grains avdp) made by placing the fruit in 1 cup of water and briefly boiling it, promotes milk-building in nursing mothers. For a decoction to be given to children, take 2–3 grams (1–$1\frac{1}{2}$ teaspoonfuls or 30.8–46.2 grains avdp) of the fruits.

CULINARY USE: Caraway has a spicy aroma and a pleasantly sharp, somewhat burning taste. Use dried whole as a schizocarp (a fruit that splits on drying), or ground.

Used in bread, cracknel, caraway sticks, salt-baked goods, fat meat dishes, cabbage and cabbage dishes, potatoes, stew, curds spread on bread, cheese-making, liqueur preparation (kümmel).

Has the property of neutralizing meat dishes, promotes digestion, stimulates the appetite, and counteracts stomach and intestinal complaints (see above).

(a) Blossom
(b) Double fruit (seed)

Caraway

WILD CARROT

SCIENTIFIC NAME: *Daucus carota.*

OTHER POPULAR NAMES: Queen Anne's lace, bee's nest plant, bird's nest root.

FAMILY: Umbelliferae—Parsley or Carrot Family.

RANGE: Wild carrot has been native to the Mediterranean region since primitive times. Today it grows wild all over Europe and Asia on dry or barren meadows, on refuse dumps and fallow land. In North America, the common wild carrot is an immigrant from Europe and is a nuisance to farmers.

DESCRIPTION: The wild carrot seeks out for itself light, silicic acid, humus-rich soil, warmth and water. This harmonious plant is one of the most valuable herbs. In the first year, the orange-tinted, sturdy root sends doubly to quadruply pinnate leaves upward. In its second year, the flowering process begins. Smaller and smaller leaves sprout on the stem up to the uppermost umbels. From below they reach up and enclose even the smallest umbellets of white blossoms, at the very top. In the middle of the umbel there is often a single, purple blossom, slightly larger than the white ones.

ELEMENTS CONTAINED: The root contains 6–12 per cent sugar, pectin, inosite, essential oil, lecithin, glutamine, phosphatide, vitamins B and C and carotin, which ordinarily is present only in the leaves, flowers and fruits of the plant. According to latest research, carotin is necessary for the reception of light energy by the plant. In the human organism, carotin yields vitamin A, in which visual purple (a pigment contained in the retina of the eye) is especially concentrated. The ashes contain silicic acid, iron and traces of arsenic, cobalt, copper and nickel.

MEDICINAL USE: The seeds—*Semen Dauci*; the fresh root—*Radix Dauci*; the thickened sap of the root—*Sucus Dauci*.

Grated wild carrot can be applied externally on burns and for the healing of ulcers. The effect of this old household remedy has now been confirmed by modern medicine. Especially, carotin dissolved in oil is an exceptional remedy for the most extensive burns, which otherwise would lead to death, as well as in cases of freezing, in which the limbs have already turned blue-black.

Used internally, the root is an effective remedy for intestinal parasites. Since some people suffer worm attacks due to fertilizing vegetables with fresh feces, grated carrot salad, steamed carrots (which lose only a little of their quality), and carrot juice should not be spared from the regular diet.

In cases of European cholera of children, the patient is given only carrot soup all day long. The root of the wild carrot is said to have a diuretic effect. The thickened sap is taken for cough and catarrh of the air passages. For stomach and intestinal troubles, fresh carrot juice is mixed with flaxseed tea or a vegetable broth. (This should consist only of root vegetables, potatoes and water. Condiments such as salt, pepper and onions should not be used.)

CULINARY USE: A country brew has long been made from wild carrots. The wild carrot and the garden carrot are classified as varieties of a single species, but the yellowish woody root of the wild carrot is very different from the succulent orange root of the garden type.

(Also see illustration, page 122)

Celandine

CELANDINE

SCIENTIFIC NAME: *Chelidonium majus.*

OTHER POPULAR NAMES: Common celandine, greater celandine, swallow-wort, tetterwort, garden celandine, great celandine, chelidonium. (Not related to lesser celandine, which belongs to the Buttercup Family.)

FAMILY: Papaveraceae—Poppy Family.

RANGE: This plant has spread over the entire world and grows on refuse dumps, along fences, walls and roads and under hedges.

DESCRIPTION: As early as January, the sturdy, perennial root-stock often sends up young leaves. Not long afterward, the ground-rosette with its soft, roundish-lobed leaves is formed. A multi-branched stem sprouts forth in the flowering process, and flower shoots spring from the axes of the leaves. Golden-yellow flowers appear and then fade away—the petals drop off as in the case of the related poppy. The long seed pods thrust themselves upward, severely erect. The taste of the plant is bitter, sharp and burning.

ELEMENTS CONTAINED: Chelidonine, homochelidonine, chelery-thrine, protopine (an opium alkaloid), sanguinarine, berberine, sparteine, an essential oil, a yellow resin and an abundance of calcium and ammonium-magnesium phosphate.

MEDICINAL USE: The whole plant—*Herba Chelidonii*; flowers—*Flores Chelidonii*; roots—*Radix Chelidonii.*

Celandine, once highly prized as a medicinal plant, for a time almost fell into oblivion, but today it has been restored to a place among herbal remedies. The root is especially effective for liver and gall-bladder conditions, while the flowers have a beneficial influence on the thyroid gland. The fresh sap applied to warts over a period of time causes them to disappear.

CULINARY USE: None.

Centaury

SCIENTIFIC NAMES: *Erythraea centaurium (Centaurium umbellatum).*

OTHER POPULAR NAMES: Christ's Ladder, feverwort, fellwort.

FAMILY: Gentianaceae—Gentian Family.

RANGE: In Europe, the centaury plant is found along forest edges, on meadows and pasturage. It prefers soil that is somewhat damp, loamy, sandy and limey. There are several native North American species of the genus *Erythraea*. However, herbalists call a related plant, *Sabatia stellaris*, American centaury, because it has uses similar to those of *E. centaurium*.

DESCRIPTION: According to Greek myth, this plant was recommended to mankind as a medicinal plant by the centaur Chiron, who was skilled in medicine. The root of this annual to biennial plant develops a rosette of elliptical leaves from which a stem with opposed, also elliptical but smaller, sharp-tipped leaves rises. The multiple-forked false umbels of pink flowers do not open until late summer. With the approach of rain-presaging air, however, they will close again, even on a clear day. The whole plant has a sharply bitter taste.

ELEMENTS CONTAINED: The most important constituent is a bitter principle glycoside, erythrocentaurin; in addition, resin, essential oil, stearine, palmitic (palmitinic) acid, magnesium lactate, mucilage, sugar, erytharin (a bitter, crystalline, colorless glycoside), ceryl alcohol, gum, wax, mineral salts.

MEDICINAL USE: The plant—*Herba Centaurii.*

Make a decoction with 1–3 grams (15.4–46.2 grains avdp) of the plant briefly boiled in 1 cup of water, and use it as a compress and wash to get beneficial effects on skin troubles.

Internally, the tea made from 1–3 grams (15.4–46.2 grains avdp) of the plant scalded with 1 cup of boiling water, is given for metabolic troubles. Liver and gall-bladder complaints, weakness of the digestive tract, loss of appetite, catarrh of the stomach, and heartburn, are all within its range of use. Centaury tea is also helpful in cases of rheumatism, gout, anemia and diabetes.

CULINARY USE: None.

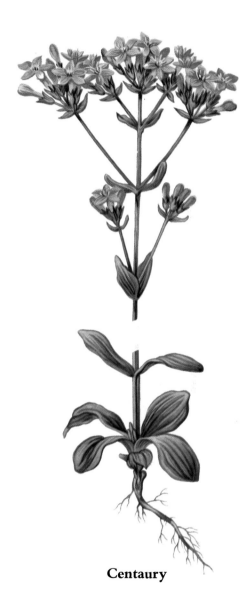

Centaury

WILD CHAMOMILE

SCIENTIFIC NAME: *Matricaria chamomilla*.

OTHER POPULAR NAMES: Sweet false camomile (chamomile), German camomile, common matricary.

FAMILY: Compositae—Composite Family.

RANGE: Chamomile loves the light. It is found on fields, fallow land, and along the edges of fields. (Indigenous to southern Europe, it covers Europe and northern Asia, and has escaped to the eastern United States and Argentina.)

DESCRIPTION: From the seeds, which are sowed in the autumn, develops first the soft, pinnate leaf rosette. This winters over and does not put forth its flowers until the following spring. Its compressed leaves appear first as nodes, then unfold into a fluffily bushy, feathery, light-green foliage.

Located above on the ends are the numerous, golden-yellow flower heads with their soft white petals. A hollow space at the bottom of the flower and the sweet, aromatic scent distinguish them clearly from the flowers of the larger but medicinally worthless corn camomile *(Anthemis arvensis)*.

ELEMENTS CONTAINED: At least 0.4 per cent essential oil (dark blue azulene), bisabolene, glycoside, a bitter principle, a mixture of fats such as ceresin (mineral wax or ozokerite), stearine, linoleic acid, and choline and apigenin (inflammation retarding agents).

MEDICINAL USE: Flowers—*Flores Chamomillae vulagris*; oil—*Oleum Chamomillae aetherium*; tincture—*Tinctura Chamomillae*.

As is well known, chamomile grows practically everywhere in Europe, and it has been demonstrated to be very valuable as a medicinal plant. Harvesting cultivated chamomile is quite difficult. From time immemorial, chamomile has been one of the principal remedies in folk medicine, since it has a healing, anti-spasmodic and inflammation restraining effect. These properties make it effective internally in cases of stomach and intestinal trouble and in acute bladder catarrh.

It is used externally as a poultice on badly healing wounds, inflamed eyes, skin and mucous membranes. Also, enemas of chamomile tea have been found to be very beneficial (1 teaspoonful scalded in 1 cup of boiling water).

In cases of head colds and inflammation of the frontal and maxillary sinuses (frontal cavities and Highmore's antrum), a chamomile steam bath is made by putting 3 tablespoonfuls of chamomile in a vessel of boiling water and inhaling the steam.

In addition to the three properties named above, latest medical research has discovered an entirely new and important property: according to this, chamomile has a decontaminating effect on the toxins of various bacteria, among others, the toxins of staphylococcus and streptococcus. The propagation of the bacteria is not prevented as it is when antibiotics are administered. In many cases, the effect of the latter is to create a resistance on the part of the bacteria, thus making the dispensed remedy ineffective. When chamomile is administered, the poisonous substances given off by the bacteria, which have an extraordinary effect on the human organism, are rendered non-injurious. Only very small quantities of chamomile essential oil are required for this. This new knowledge also now explains why the general condition of a patient so quickly improves after the use of chamomile.

CULINARY USE: Some people like a weak blend of Chamomile tea as refreshment.

(See illustration, page 7)

CHERVIL

SCIENTIFIC NAME: *Anthriscus cerefolium.*

OTHER POPULAR NAME: Salad chervil.

FAMILY: Umbelliferae—Parsley or Carrot Family.

RANGE: Chervil is native to Europe, but has been naturalized in parts of North America.

DESCRIPTION: From the tapering root-stock a many-branched hairy stem grows to a height of 1–2 feet (30–60 cm). The leaves are very finely divided and the white florets are clustered in small umbels. The entire plant exudes a scent closely resembling that of anise. The plant is a biennial, but is grown as an annual.

ELEMENTS CONTAINED: Volatile oil, glycoside, apiin.

MEDICINAL USE: The entire plant is dried and used externally on bruises and local tumors. Is a mild diuretic and aids metabolism and uterine functions.

CULINARY USE: Chervil leaves are used in salads and soups, and are especially good in potato salad. The leaves should be picked when young, like parsley, and can be frozen. Chervil is one of the basic herbs, along with chives and parsley, of the culinary seasoning mixture called *fines herbes*.

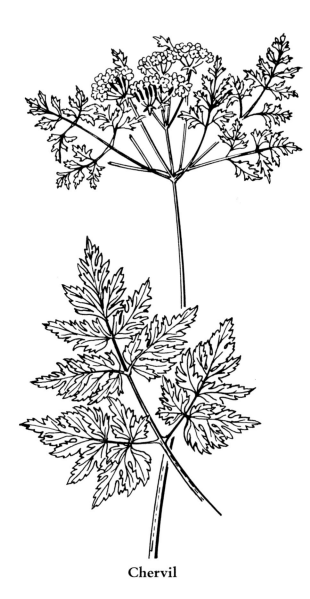

Chervil

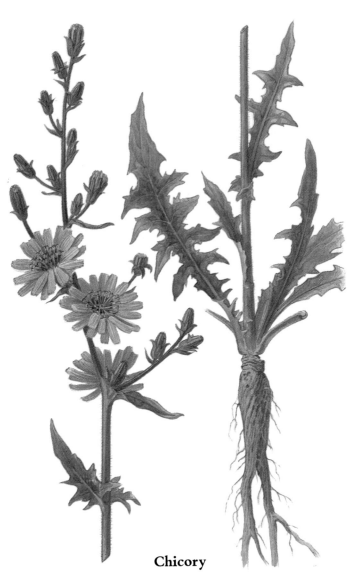

Chicory

CHICORY

SCIENTIFIC NAME: *Cichorium intybus*.

OTHER POPULAR NAMES: Succory, endive.

FAMILY: Compositae—Composite Family.

RANGE: Roads, field borders, waste land and barren meadows with dry soil are the places in Europe and in the temperate region of Asia, where chicory is native. It has become thoroughly naturalized in the United States.

DESCRIPTION: Chicory has a long, fleshy root full of a milky sap. Above ground a leaf rosette develops very similar to that of the related dandelion, but more compact. The tough branched stalk is hard to break, as anyone tempted to pick the light blue flowers will find. The flowers face eastwards toward the rising sun and by afternoon become withered and faded, to be replaced the next morning by newly opened flowers. Chicory, although a composite, has only ray flowers—the disc flowers are entirely lacking. All summer long, an inexhaustible supply of flowers opens.

ELEMENTS CONTAINED: In the milky sap, bitter principles (cichoriin and intybin), fat, mannite (mannitol), and latex are present. The root contains a great deal of inulin. Analysis of the flowers yields a glycoside, cichoriin. The ashes of chicory contain potassium oxide, silicic acid, magnesium oxide, sodium oxide, and some iron oxide.

MEDICINAL USE: The root—*Radix Cichorii*; leaves and flowers—*Folia cum Flores Cichorii*.

Only wild chicory is suitable for medicinal purposes. For external use, a decoction is prepared of 2–4 grams (30.8–61.6 grains avdp) of the root boiled for 3 minutes in 1 cup of water, which is used for compresses in cases of eye inflammation.

Internally, the tea of flowers and leaves made from 2–4 grams (30.8–61.6 grains avdp) scalded with 1 cup of boiling water, is effective on the liver and the gall bladder. This important liver remedy attends to the flow of bile, helps in cases of icterus (jaundice), gallstones, obstruction of the digestive organs with mucus, dyspepsia (a form of indigestion), loss of appetite, and congestion of the liver. Also, blood-building is stimulated, as well as formation of the substances of bones, muscles and nerves.

CULINARY USE: The roots of chicory have long been roasted and ground in Europe for use as a coffee substitute or to give added strength and bitterness to real coffee. The young roots and leaves are used in salads—especially the blanched leaves of the variety of chicory called Endive or Witloof. In Belgium especially, the roots are boiled and served with butter.

Endives may be pureed, dipped in batter and deep-fried, browned in butter, braised, put in soufflés, or simmered and served with a variety of sauces (Béchamel, Mornay, Velouté).

CHIVE

SCIENTIFIC NAME: *Allium schoenoprasum*.
OTHER POPULAR NAME: Chive garlic.
FAMILY: Liliaceae—Lily Family.
RANGE: Native to Europe and northern Asia, but naturalized in North America, especially in the region of Lakes Superior and Huron.
DESCRIPTION: The genus *Allium* includes the onion, leek, garlic, shallot and other plants with a characteristic pungent aroma. The chive, which is easily grown in a window box, can reach a height of about 1 foot (30 cm) from a cluster of small bulbs beneath the soil. Outdoor plants may be potted and brought indoors for the winter. The long, tubular green leaves surround the blue-green flower stems, each of which ends in a globe-like head of dull, pale-purple flowers.
ELEMENTS CONTAINED: Proteins, minerals, high vitamin C content, fair amount of vitamin B, carotin, iron, arsenic.
MEDICINAL USE: The chive, being much more delicate than onion and garlic, has not figured in the official pharmacopoeia. Garlic, in particular, has value as a diaphoretic, diuretic and expectorant, and along with onion is much used to treat chills and colds. Chives stimulate the appetite, aid digestion, help lower blood pressure and combat anemia, however.
CULINARY USE: The delicate, oniony taste of chives makes them useful in many dishes where onion and garlic would be too strong. Chives should not be dried but may be frozen or put in vinegar.

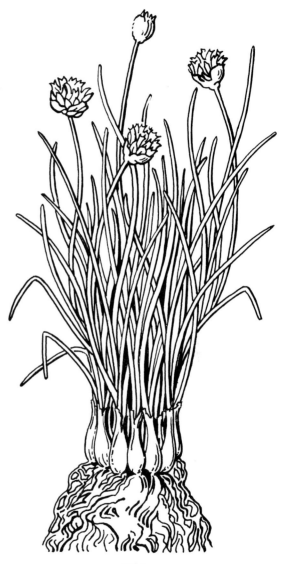

Chive

Red Clover

SCIENTIFIC NAME: *Trifolium pratense.*

OTHER POPULAR NAMES: Purple clover, wild clover, wild red clover.

FAMILY: Leguminosae—Pea or Pulse Family.

RANGE: The oldest information on the cultivation of field clovers goes back to the time of the Spanish rulership over the Netherlands. Today, it is cultivated throughout entire central Europe the same as white clover *(Trifolium alba)*, and naturalized in the United States.

DESCRIPTION: The well-known trifoliate leaves spring upward from the root on a long stem up to 60 cm (2 feet) tall and swing out over the earth. White clover creeps, but the red variety does not. Even in ancient times, the superstition was current that it would bring good luck in gaming as well as in living. Whoever carried such a triple leaf clover about with him possessed the gift of being able to detect witches, sorcerers, and good fairies. Christianity saw in the 3-part leaf a symbol of the Trinity. Hence the ground-plan of churches and church windows were designed after the cloverleaf. The inflorescence of this species of clover is shaped like a ball. Petals and stamen are grown together in one piece. Children like to pluck out the single blossoms on the meadows and suck the sweet juice out of them.

ELEMENTS CONTAINED: Essential oil, tannin, perfume, nitrogen, sodium.

MEDICINAL USE: The flowers—*Flores Trifolii rubri.*

Red- and white-clover blossoms are a popular cough remedy. White-clover blossoms were in popular use in folk medicine against gout, rheumatism, and leucorrhea (vaginal discharge). The texture of fingernails and toenails will improve from partaking of gentle clover tea. Pour $\frac{1}{4}$ litre ($\frac{1}{2}$ pint) of boiling water over 28 grams (1 oz avdp) of the leaves.

CULINARY USE: Blooms make a good country wine. American Indians of the western United States are said to eat red clover raw as a salad, but others who have tried it found it hard to digest.

(a) Blossom (enlarged)

Red Clover

Colt's Foot

SCIENTIFIC NAME: *Tussilago farfara.*

OTHER POPULAR NAMES: Coughwort, foal's foot, horse hoof, horse foot, bull's foot, ginger root.

FAMILY: Compositae—Composite Family.

RANGE: Throughout Europe, Asia and North Africa, colt's foot loves damp loam, lime-containing soils, found on slopes, road-sides and railway embankments. It has also been naturalized all over eastern North America.

DESCRIPTION: In the first sun of spring, the perennial root-stock, which constantly sends forth rooting runners, sends a scaly stalk upward, bearing a glowing yellow flower. The flowers are very much dependent on the sun—they close up at night and when the sky is overcast. Not until after the blooming period does the plant fully complete its cycle and send up its long-stemmed, roundish leaves that are white beneath, from a basal rosette of leaves.

ELEMENTS CONTAINED: Inulin, tannin, traces of essential oil, xanthophyll, mucilage. If there are metals in the soil, the plant absorbs them.

MEDICINAL USE: Blossoms—*Flores Farfarae*; leaves—*Folia Farfarae*.

The fresh leaves, after being rolled with a rolling pin to crush the veins, are used externally in cases of inflammation, leg sores, and ulcers. In cases of fever, Kneipp laid the leaves on the breast, but also locally and in cases of the disease manifestations described above. A decoction alleviates scrofulous ulcers as well as disease of the conjunctiva (mucous membrane lining the eyelids) and the edges of the eyelids.

A tea made from 5–10 grams (77–154 grains avdp) of the leaves and flowers scalded with a cup of boiling water, is used as a cough remedy, in cases of bronchial catarrh, hoarseness and clogging of the breathing passages with mucus.

CULINARY USE: None.

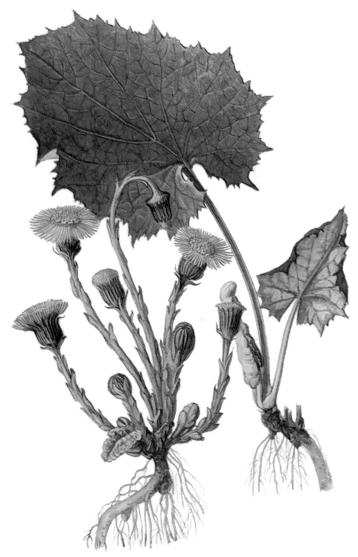

Colt's Foot

COLUMBINE

SCIENTIFIC NAME: *Aquilegia vulgaris.*

OTHER POPULAR NAMES: European columbine, common columbine.

FAMILY: Ranunculaceae—Crowfoot or Buttercup Family.

RANGE: Specimens of this plant occur singly in the shade of trees and bushes growing in the wild, but are more often found in gardens. A native of Europe, *Aquilegia vulgaris*, has been naturalized in North America. There are also several native species in America.

DESCRIPTION: This esteemed plant has large divided leaves growing in sets of three on a stem. These are dull green on the upper surface but are blue-green on the underside, and downy. The downward-hanging, large blossoms of the columbine growing in the wild are blue to violet, while the garden columbine is whitish-blue or yellowish-red.

ELEMENTS CONTAINED: The plant when in flower contains substances yielding prussic acid, and, in addition, oil and mucilage. The plant has a narcotic effect and is disagreeably sharp and bitter tasting.

MEDICINAL USE: The whole plant is used—called *Herba Aquilegiae* in pharmacy. Columbine is used externally on fistulas. Internally, the pressed-out juice of the fresh plant is given for chronic skin eruptions and in the treatment of external fistulas. Columbine is also effective against swelling of the spleen or liver, jaundice, colic-like abdominal pains and dropsy. Because of the plant's prussic acid content and its narcotic effect, let your physician prescribe the proper dosage.

CULINARY USE: None.

Columbine

COMMON COMFREY

SCIENTIFIC NAME: *Symphytum officinale.*

OTHER POPULAR NAMES: Cumfrey, healing herb, blackwort, bruisewort, wallwort, gum plant.

FAMILY: Boraginaceae—Borage Family.

RANGE: Comfrey is found practically everywhere in Europe and northern Asia and has been naturalized in North America. Found in damp meadows, on banks of streams, and by wet ditches and ponds.

DESCRIPTION: From a sturdy root, the stalk climbs to a height of a metre (about 40 inches). Its alternate leaves are pointed, lanceolate (lance-shaped) and coarsely hairy. From the upper axils spiral inflorescences gradually unfold, on which violet, less often white, bell-shaped blossoms develop.

ELEMENTS CONTAINED: The root contains mucilage, starch, gum, sugar, resin, some essential oil, asparagine, allantoin, and silicic acid. The blossoms and the plant contain alkaloids in smaller traces, which have a paralyzing effect on the central nervous system.

MEDICINAL USE: The root—*Radix Symphyti.*

The comfrey root is mainly used externally on wounds, bruises and abscesses of long standing. This medicinal appears to work especially on the periosteum, benefitting bone diseases and fractures. A powder manufactured from the root is used to stanch the flow of blood from recent wounds.

For internal use, a tea is prepared, 20 grams (308 grains avdp = 5/7 oz) of the chopped root scalded by pouring over it $\frac{1}{2}$ litre (about 17 ounces) of boiling water. The plentiful mucilage content is effective against diarrhea, catarrh of the mucous membranes of the bronchial tubes, stomach and intestinal bleeding (hemorrhages), and dysentery.

CULINARY USE: As a pot-herb, comfrey can be used for greens if the cooking water is discarded and replaced with fresh water, which is then brought to a boil. This removes irritants from the leaves.

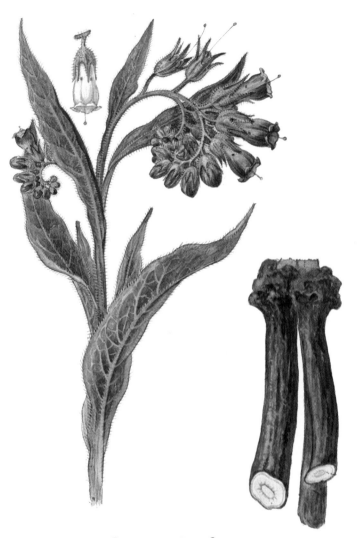

Common Comfrey

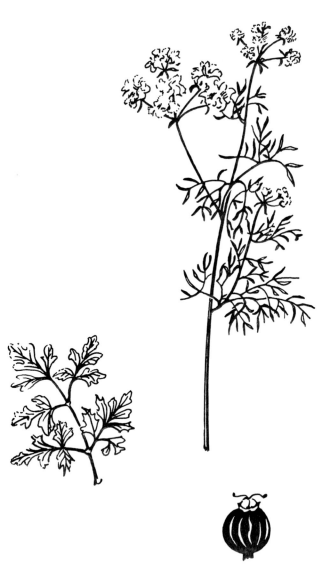

Coriander

CORIANDER

SCIENTIFIC NAME: *Coriandrum sativum*.

OTHER POPULAR NAMES: Common coriander, coriander seed herb.

FAMILY: Umbelliferae—Parsley or Carrot Family.

RANGE: Coriander is native to southern Europe and Asia Minor. The early Israelites, the Egyptians and the Romans were acquainted with it. It is nowadays cultivated in gardens in England and Europe, as well as the United States (where it is sometimes found as a weed). The seeds are sowed either in September or April for harvesting the following August.

DESCRIPTION: Coriander grows a slim, erect, hollow stem to a height of 25 cm–1 m (1–2 or even 3 feet). The plant has a strong smell. The bipinnate leaves are divided into narrowly linear segments, the lower leaves being deeply cut. The small, white flowers grow in compound umbels. The petals of the outer flowers of each umbel are enlarged like rays. The green seed (which is really the fruit) has an unpleasant smell and taste, but turns pleasantly aromatic on maturation.

ELEMENTS CONTAINED: An essential oil called coriander oil or coriandrol, consisting mainly of linool.

MEDICINAL USE: The fruits—*Fructus Coriandri.*

Coriander is used medicinally as a stomachic and a carminative (inducing gas expulsion) agent, and for intestinal complaints.

CULINARY USE: Coriander seeds (as the fruits are called) are used as an ingredient of hot curries and sauces. The young leaves and shoots are used to spice stews, soups and salads. The aroma is not very pleasant, but the taste is pleasantly spicy. Fresh: Not usable. Dried: Pulverize with mortar and pestle or grind.

Coriander seed is used in bread, Christmas baked goods, preparation of sausages, meat dishes, with red beets, in plum jam, cabbage dishes, sauces, and in the preparation of herb liqueurs.

Cornflower

SCIENTIFIC NAME: *Centaurea cyanis.*

OTHER POPULAR NAMES: Bachelor's button, bluebottle, corn bluebottle, common cornflower, cyani.

FAMILY: Compositae—Composite Family.

RANGE: The cornflower is native to the Mediterranean region and its habitat reaches from Sicily, over the Balkans, and on into the Middle East. It has been spread over the entire world with the cultivation of grain.

DESCRIPTION: On a stem about 70 cm ($27\frac{1}{2}$ inches) high, which is thickly branched and bears narrow leaves, stand the composite flowers with large, 6-pointed, ray blossoms and many smaller disc flowers in great quantities.

ELEMENTS CONTAINED: Tannin, blue pigment.

MEDICINAL USE: The blossoms—*Flores Cyani.*

The flowers are used in tea mixtures practically exclusively for coloration. Here and there, the cornflower has been known as a folk remedy for leucorrhea (vaginal discharge) and as a purgative. For tea, 2–4 grams (30.8–61.6 grains avdp) of dried flowers are scalded with 1 cup boiling water.

CULINARY USE: None.

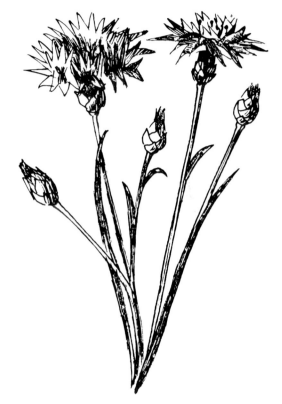

Cornflower

Cowslip

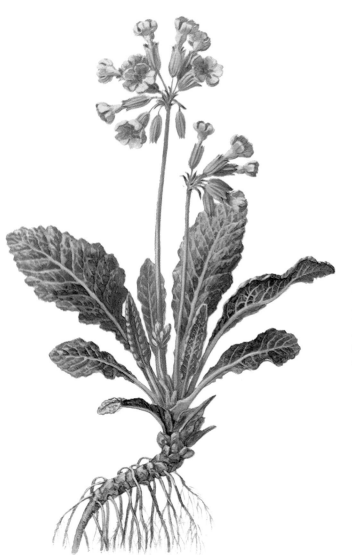

Cowslip

SCIENTIFIC NAMES: *Primula officinalis (P. veris)*.

OTHER POPULAR NAMES: Primrose, paigle, fairy cup, petty mullein, oxlip, butter rose, English cowslip.

FAMILY: Primulaceae—Primrose Family.

RANGE: In central Europe, this spring flower grows strewn over meadows, slopes, and in light woods. (The American cowslip is a totally different plant of the Buttercup Family).

DESCRIPTION: The short, brown root-stock sends up a leaf rosette of wrinkled leaves, the undersides of which are velvety-haired, out of which climbs the brief, leafless stem to end in an umbel, of which the golden-yellow blossom, a little reddish at the base, bends shyly to one side.

ELEMENTS CONTAINED: A glycoside: primulaverin, which is split by an enzyme, also present.

MEDICINAL USE: The blossoms—*Flores Primulae*; the leaves—*Folia Primulae*; the roots—*Radix Primulae*.

Externally, a decoction of the root from 1 gram (15.4 grains avdp) slightly boiled in 1 cup of water, is used as a bath for rheumatism, contusions and wounds. The tea made from 2–4 grams (30.8–61.6 grains avdp) of all three parts of the plant scalded with 1 cup of boiling water, is very good for loosening phlegm and as an expectorant, for which reason it aids in cases of colds and bronchial catarrh.

CULINARY USE: The flowers are distilled to make a country wine.

ENGLISH DAISY

SCIENTIFIC NAME: *Bellis perennis.*

OTHER POPULAR NAMES: Daisy, common daisy, true daisy.

FAMILY: Compositae—Composite Family.

RANGE: The daisy grows practically everywhere throughout central Europe, in meadows, field borders, and village commons. It is rarely found in North America outside of gardens, although, its cousin, the ox-eye daisy (actually a chrysanthemum) has been widely naturalized there.

DESCRIPTION: While the meadows are still wet with melted snow, one morning thousands of tiny, white stars may be found winking among the grasses. In the middle of each flower is a round, convex disc, filled with the gold of the sun. One may not have noticed their growth before, and yet each stands already open in the midst of a leaf-rosette of small, oval leaves, on a slender, leafless stem. Their composite blossoms have golden yellow, tubular disc-flowers and white or reddish ray flowers. Demure yet striking to the eye, they decorate the meadows of Europe practically all year round. Even at New Year's time, they still remain on snow-free sunny meadows.

ELEMENTS CONTAINED: Saponin, tannin, resin, essential oil, sugar, mucilage, protein, a bitter principle, malic, tartaric, acetic, and oxalic acid; fat oil.

MEDICINAL USE: Flowers—*Flores Bellidis.*

The daisy is very good for the liver. In the spring, when few other herbs are available, the entire plant with its blossoms can be chopped up fine and mixed with lettuce or curds. Daily use over a period of a few weeks brings about purification of the blood. It also has a loosening effect on mucus in the air passages, particularly the bronchial tubes.

CULINARY USE: None.

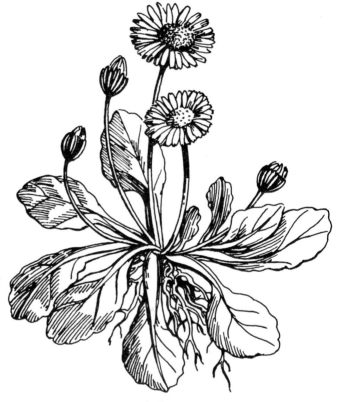

English Daisy

DANDELION

SCIENTIFIC NAMES: *Taraxacum officinale (T. dens-leonis* and *Leontodon taraxacum).*

OTHER POPULAR NAMES: Blow ball, cankerwort, common dandelion, lion's tooth, dent-de-lion, wet-a-bed, piss-en-lit.

FAMILY: Compositae—Composite Family.

RANGE: The dandelion has spread throughout the northern hemisphere and even into the far north. It grows everywhere in meadows, fields and ditches, on slopes and in yards and gardens as a weed.

DESCRIPTION: The stake-like root bores deep into the earth. Above ground, it sends forth a rosette of many leaves. The most valuable plants, found especially in the mountains, where they receive a great deal of light, show a deeply incised leaf, often as deep as the middle rib. Plants growing in damp shade are less toothed and many times are even entirely undivided.

Another sign also bears evidence to the fact that the dandelion has a very special relationship with the sun. The composite flower head reared aloft on its long, smooth, hollow stem—an image of the sun itself—exhibits its golden fullness of flower only in the sunshine. Along comes a cloud and the whole flower crown disappears, enclosed in its green calyx. This sunny inflorescence develops into a whole world of stars, known to every child as a "blow ball." The white, milky sap of the stems can have a slightly poisonous effect on children.

ELEMENTS CONTAINED: Choline, a bitter principle, starch, saponin, fat, enzyme, traces of essential oil, wax, mucilage, levuline, carotinoids; several vitamins, among them especially Vitamin B_2; silicic acid, potassium, magnesium, copper, zinc, caoutchouc. The mixture of contents changes with the seasons.

MEDICINAL USE: The root—*Radix Taraxaci*; the plant—*Herba Taraxaci.*

Today, the dandelion is one of our most important medicinal plants. The young spring leaves are used in a blood-purification course of treatment. Two wide ranges of effect can be distinguished. There is first the mild stimulation of the large elimination organs of the organism, the liver and the kidneys. To expel stones caught in the ureter, the patient drinks daily a whole litre (quart) of dandelion tea made from 2–4 grams (30.8–61.6 grains avdp) scalded, per 1 cup of boiling water. To prevent renewal of stone formation, the treatment is continued at weekly intervals. Dandelion tea is also taken to stimulate liver and gall-bladder activity.

The second field of use is rheumatism. For this, 1 teaspoonful of the plant is taken in 1 cup of water, either scalded or boiled for a brief time. The tea is allowed to steep for 10 minutes before straining. The patient is to drink one cup at a time, every morning and noon. Also, the freshly squeezed juice, which can be bought at a health food store or a pharmacy, is given morning and noon, 1–2 tablespoonfuls at a time in 1 cup of warm water. Such a course of dandelion treatment, carried on for 4–6 weeks, has an especially beneficial effect on chronic arthrosis (arthrosis deformans), as well as on degenerative disease of the vertebral articulation (spandulosis deformans).

CULINARY USE: In France and Italy, dandelions are sold as greens on the market and are especially popular in salads in those countries. As a cooked vegetable use leaves either cultivated or gathered wild. Wash thoroughly and cut each leaf off with a knife, then leave in sink to "bleed" its milky sap (which gives a bitter taste). Wash again before cooking. The roots have been used as a coffee substitute, and a popular country wine is also made from dandelion. For good plants, seeds can be purchased.

(See illustration, page 4)

Dead Nettle

SCIENTIFIC NAME: *Lamium album*.

OTHER POPULAR NAMES: White dead nettle, blind nettle, stingless nettle, white nettle, white archangel.

FAMILY: Labiatae—Mint Family.

RANGE: The dead nettle is widespread throughout the cool part of Europe. It grows along roadsides, on meadows, along fences and the edges of woods, under hedges and on rubbish dumps. *L. maculatum*, the spotted dead nettle, is naturalized in the eastern United States.

DESCRIPTION: With its sturdy leaf structure, the dead nettle really does have something nettle-like about it. The large, white flowers sit like false-whorls around the leaf axes. The upper lip of the flower is arched like a helmet; the underlip is triple-lobed. On the snowy white are found yellow spots. Blooming period is from April to October and even beyond.

ELEMENTS CONTAINED: A great deal of mucilage; tannin, essential oil, an alkaloid (coniine); saponin is obtained from the roots to the flowers.

MEDICINAL USE: The flower without its calyx—*Flores Lamii albi*, or *Flores Lamii*; the entire plant—*Herba cum Radix Lamii*.

Make the tea from 1 teaspoonful scalded with 1 cup of boiling water. Tea-drenched cloth compresses are laid on ulcers, varicose veins, and swollen glands; in addition, the tea is used for suppressing earache. Dead nettle tea has a phlegm-loosening, soothing, inflammation-preventing effect and is especially beneficial to the female genital tract. Also beneficially influences kidney troubles, catarrh of the stomach and intestines, and inflammation of the air passages.

CULINARY USE: The young flower tips can be gently sauteed in butter for use as a vegetable.

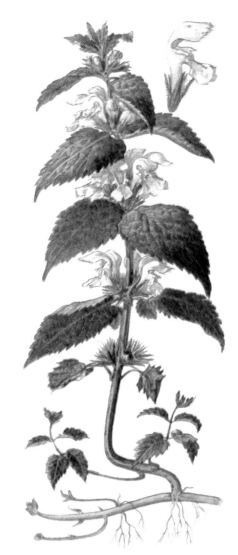

Dead Nettle

43

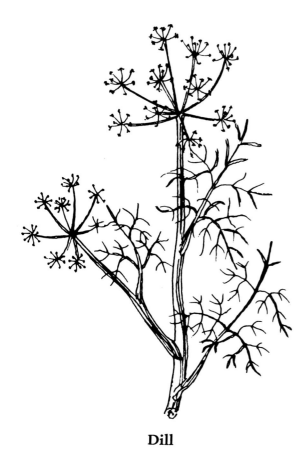

Dill

DILL

SCIENTIFIC NAME: *Anethum graveolens.*

OTHER POPULAR NAME: Dillweed.

FAMILY: Umbelliferae—Parsley or Carrot Family.

RANGE: Dill is native to the Middle East and Europe and is naturalized in North America. It was well known to the early Egyptians and Hebrews as a seasoning and medicinal plant. The first monks to enter central Europe probably brought it along with them. Today, dill is raised everywhere in gardens, but it also grows wild.

DESCRIPTION: This annual plant has a spindle-shaped root and grows quickly to a height of 50–125 cm (19–49 inches). The leaves are lightly pinnate. From the ends of the stems arch large, abundantly radiating umbels of yellow blossoms.

ELEMENTS CONTAINED: 2.5–4 per cent essential oil is the most important constituent; and up to 18 per cent fat oil.

MEDICINAL USE: The fruits—*Fructus Anethi.*

In medicine, the plant is used to promote the formation of milk in nursing mothers. It aids diuresis and menstruation and is also carminative and antispasmodic.

It has a digestion-promoting effect. Tea: 1 teaspoonful, over which pour 1 cupful of boiling water. Promotes sleep, counters flatulence and nausea.

CULINARY USE: Dill is used to spice sauces, fish dishes, salads and cucumbers and is used in making dill pickles.

Dill has a very pleasant, spicy aroma, which is brought out if one simply soaks or steeps the fresh plant—but does not let it cook (boil). When used fresh, dill should be chopped fine. When dried, use in powdered form—the dill seed can be ground to powder in a mortar with salt.

Use dill in soups, sauces, vegetables, salads (especially cucumber and tomato salad), for preserving, with mutton and in stewed dishes, with fish, in herb butter, with eggs, curd dishes and marinades.

ELECAMPANE

SCIENTIFIC NAME: *Inula helenium*.

OTHER POPULAR NAMES: Scabwort, elf dock, velvet dock, inula, horse-heal, elf-wort.

FAMILY: Compositae—Composite Family.

RANGE: Elecampane probably hails from central Asia, then entered Europe from Asia Minor and has been grown in European gardens as a medicinal and kitchen herb for many centuries. It grows wild today on damp meadows in many parts of Europe and is widely naturalized in eastern North America.

DESCRIPTION: From the sturdy, branched root-stock grows a straight, breast-high stalk with many wide, oval, undivided leaves with pointed ends, and coarsely saw-toothed. The stem branches out at the top and ends in a cluster of flowers resembling those of arnica (early botanists called the plant "false arnica"). A long-haired pappus tuft crowns the fruit, and there are no paleae (scales on the receptacle of plants of the Composite Family).

ELEMENTS CONTAINED: In the autumn, the root-stock contains a great deal of inulin, alantol, up to 3 per cent essential oils, helenin, acantholactone and some azulene.

MEDICINAL USE: The root—*Radix Helenii*—is used.

A decoction of 2–4 grams (30.8–61.6 grains avdp) of the root is used externally for skin diseases, mainly as an antiseptic.

Internal doses have a stimulating effect on digestion, and have a diuretic effect on catarrhal conditions of the bladder and urethra. It also promotes the flow of bile. Elecampane works as an expectorant in the air passages in chronic bronchitis and whooping cough. In certain forms of tuberculosis, it encourages the healing process.

CULINARY USE: Elecampane is sometimes used as an aromatic in making beer.

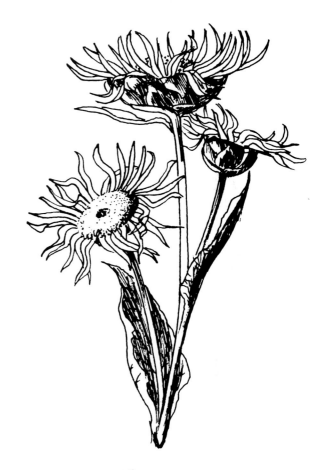

Elecampane

45

EYEBRIGHT

SCIENTIFIC NAME: *Euphrasia officinalis.*
OTHER POPULAR NAMES: Euphrasy, euphrasia.
FAMILY: Scrophulariaceae—Figwort Family.
RANGE: Eyebright is found throughout central Europe in meadows, on dry slopes, in forests and in the mountains as well as in the lowlands.
DESCRIPTION: Anyone climbing a mountain slope in late summer often sees this charming little plant, at most a hand-length tall, peering out from among the grass. It has small leaves that are stemless, roundish and sharply saw-toothed on the edges. In comparison to the entire plant, the flowers are oversized, usually snow white with a yellow throat.
ELEMENTS CONTAINED: Glycoside, essential oils, resin, wax, a bitter principle, tannic acid, sugar, salts.
MEDICINAL USE: The whole plant—*Herba Euphrasiae.*

As indicated by its name, eyebright since ancient times has been a good and well known remedy for eye conditions such as inflammation of the edge of the eyelid, conjunctivitis, undue sensitivity to light, weak vision, and mattering (discharge of pus) of the eyes. For external treatment, boil a teaspoonful of the dried plant in $\frac{1}{2}$ litre (about 17 oz) for a few minutes, then strain.

For internal use, either take 1 cup of the same decoction as above and sip at intervals throughout the day, or scald a teaspoonful of the dried plant with $\frac{1}{4}$ litre (about $8\frac{1}{2}$ oz) of water. The tea when drunk not only backs up the external treatment, but also beneficially affects the basic cause of the trouble, for eye complaints often have a scrofulous condition as a cause. Eyebright is also very good for the mucous membranes of the throat, the digestive organs and the lungs. However, the medicine must be given in the recommended small dosage, as it otherwise can have a poisonous effect.
CULINARY USE: None.

Eyebright

FENNEL

SCIENTIFIC NAME: *Foeniculum vulgare* (or *Foeniculum officinale*).
OTHER POPULAR NAMES: Stinking fennel, evil-smelling fennel, common fennel, wild fennel, sweet fennel, large fennel.
FAMILY: Umbelliferae—Parsley or Carrot Family.
RANGE: This vegetable, seasoning, and medicinal plant was already known at the time of the ancient Egyptians and Greeks. It is native to the Mediterranean region and today it is cultivated all over, where long, warm summers and dry autumns prevail.
DESCRIPTION: In the first year, only the root and the basic foliage are developed from the seed. The leaves, however, are already extremely pinnate and thread-thin. The broad leaf-sheathes develop a bulb-like thickening—this is the well known, aromatic fennel-vegetable. In the following year, the plant flings its inflorescence to the height of a human, sturdy umbels and umbellets in bright, gleaming yellow and without its spathes or leaf sheaths. The fruits are large, with a spicy taste. The roots do not lose their strength entirely and can last for several years.
ELEMENTS CONTAINED: The fruits contain 2–6 per cent essential oil and their ashes 3 per cent silicic acid and 2 per cent iron oxide. In the essential oil, there is 50–60 per cent anethole (anis camphor). Fennel also contains fat oil, sugar, starch, nitrogen-containing compounds, and minerals.
MEDICINAL USE: The fruits—*Fructus Foeniculi*; the plant—*Herba Foeniculi*; the straw—*Stramentum Foeniculi*; the oil—*Oleum Foeniculi*.

Fennel has a regulative effect on the digestive tract and the lactiferous (milk-producing) glands. Its carminative, anti-convulsive, and pain-relieving properties recommend it as a sedative for small children in the form of fennel honey *(Mel Foeniculi)*. It improves digestion and has a diuretic effect. Its mucus-countering and anti-convulsive properties make it helpful in cases of cough and persistent bronchitis. For children, a tea is prepared from 1–1.5 grams (15.4–23 grains avdp) and for adults, from 2–4 grams (30.8–61.6 grains avdp) of the fruit and 1 cup of water. Let it briefly boil up. Plant and straw (the cut, dried and threshed whole plant) are used only for poultices and baths.
CULINARY USE: Anise-like, it has a sweetly spicy aroma and taste. The grains are used whole or ground. Used in bread, bakery goods, Italian soups, sauces, fish dishes, salads and marinades.

Fennel

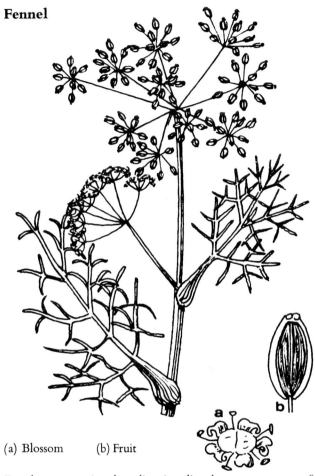

(a) Blossom   (b) Fruit

Drunk as a tea, it calms digestive disturbances—1 teaspoonful scalded by pouring a cup of hot water over it.

A southern European *Var. dulce*, Florence Foeniculum or Finocchio, has its spathes or leaf bases swollen into a bulb-like vegetable, which is blanched and eaten like celery. *Var. piperitum*, called carosella, provides food in the form of young stems. One species is grown for the leaves and aromatic seeds, which are used in seasonings.

Male Fern

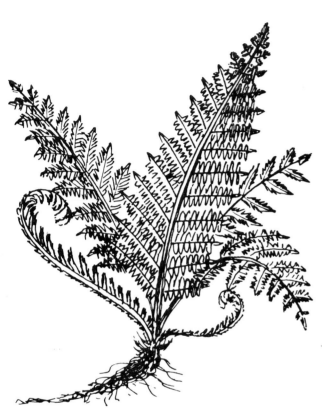

(a) Pinnate part with fruit spores.

Male Fern

SCIENTIFIC NAMES: *Aspidium filix-mas (Dryopteris filix-mas).*
OTHER POPULAR NAMES: Wood fern, shield fern, fern, aspidium, filixmas.
FAMILY: Polypodiaceae—Common Fern Family.
RANGE: In shady woods, along the stony banks of streams, in ravines, on slopes—this fern grows practically everywhere in the northern hemisphere of our planet.
DESCRIPTION: The externally brown, internally green, root-stock projects somewhat out of the ground, surrounded by rootlets that have died off and the remains of leaf stems, by way of a felt-like cocoon. Above it unfolds a lovely cluster of pinnate leaves, which at first are still rolled up and hidden away under fallen leaves, and then unroll in the spring. On the undersides of the leaves are kidney-shaped membranes, the spores (sporangia). In dry weather, the wind plays the part of seed-sower and opens up the spore capsules.
ELEMENTS CONTAINED: An acid, tannin, starch, sugar and fat oil.
MEDICINAL USE: The root-stock—*Rhizoma Filicis.*

The effective constituent of this plant, the acid, thorough investigation has proved, has a paralyzing effect on the smooth muscular system of worms, especially that of tapeworms and hook-worms. In prolonged doses, they will even kill these worms. The advantages of using this plant on human beings derive from the fact that the medicinal constituents are absorbed very slowly through the walls of the intestines and that the herb is effective against worms in a concentration that does not produce symptoms of poisoning in the human system. However, if male fern remains too long in the intestines, it is absorbed by the organism, which could damage the liver. Larger dosage leads to paralyzation of the nerves and muscles, with a following consequence of death. Loss of sight has also been observed.

For this reason, after taking male fern, which is available at the druggist's in gelatine capsules, a laxative should be taken to achieve a complete emptying of the bowels. Such treatment should be carried out only after consultation with a physician.
CULINARY USE: The young shoots of the male fern are edible and can be boiled in salted water and then tossed in butter or simmered in cream or stock.

FOXGLOVE

SCIENTIFIC NAME: *Digitalis purpurea.*

OTHER POPULAR NAMES: Digitalis, purple foxglove, fairy glove, finger flower, elves-gloves, Our-Lady's-gloves, bloody fingers, deadmen's-bells, common foxglove, American foxglove, lion's mouth, fairy fingers.

FAMILY: Scrophulariaceae—Figwort Family.

RANGE: Foxglove occurs throughout Europe and Asia in the uplands, in clearings and on stony forest slopes, and has been naturalized on the Pacific Coast of North America. It prefers primitive rock. A species occurs in European gardens with blossoms that are larger and less hairy. However, it possesses only about half the effective elements contained in the wild plant.

DESCRIPTION: In the spring a rosette of leaves grows from a cluster of roots. The stalk develops straight upward from this in summer. The large, roundish, wrinkled, lanceolate leaves are located around the stem in 3/8-arrangement. The upper part of the approximately 1 metre (40 inch) high plant produces the funnel-shaped, purple, red or white flowers.

ELEMENTS CONTAINED: 2 poisonous glycosides: digitalin and digitoxin.

MEDICINAL USE: Leaves—*Folia Digitalis*; extract—*Extractum Digitalis*; alcohol extract from the leaves—*Tinctura Digitalis*.

The strongly poisonous effect of the plant was probably known to folk medicine, since, insofar as we know today, it was used only externally in cases of goiter and glandular swelling. It was not until 1775 that the English physician Withering, of Birmingham, discovered that the tea infusion of the leaves was an exceptional remedy for dropsy. However, the poisonous properties induced him to use the remedy only on poor people! Charles Darwin's grandfather, one of the most famous physicians of his time, persuaded Withering to treat well-to-do people also with digitalis. Since then, the reputation of the remedy grew from year to year and is still retained today.

Relaxation of the myocardium (a muscle of the heart) and defects of the cardiac valve were treated with digitalis. The remedies in homeopathy which contain substances from foxglove are dispensed for cases of circulatory trouble, dropsy of the peritoneum, and all heart conditions. Digitalis contains strong poisons, of which digitoxin has the strongest effect. For this reason, it is to be taken only on prescription by a physician. Even very small doses can lead to death.

CULINARY USE: None.

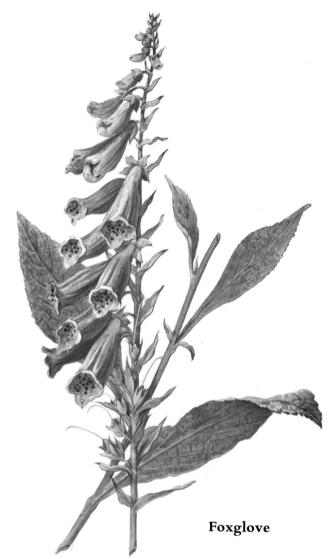

Foxglove

Yellow Gentian

Yellow Gentian

SCIENTIFIC NAME: *Gentiana lutea*.

OTHER POPULAR NAMES: Gentian, bitter-root, bitter-wort.

FAMILY: Gentianaceae—Gentian Family.

RANGE: In Europe, the yellow gentian grows mainly in the Alps to a height of 2,500 m (8,200 feet), also in the Lower Alps, in the Black Forest, and in the mountainous region of the Swabian Alb, and in the mountain areas throughout middle and southern Europe and eastward to Asia Minor.

DESCRIPTION: The outstanding aspect of the yellow gentian is its root growth. The powerful root, striking deep into the ground and lasting for decades, has a rosette of leaves which grows above ground in the spring and provides the chlorophyll needed for growth. This picture remains unchanged for 7 years, then abruptly a powerful stalk shoots up, with oval leaves in pairs. In the upper third of the stalk, the leaves grow smaller, and surround the golden yellow flowers.

ELEMENTS CONTAINED: Up to 3.5 per cent bitter principle glycoside; a special kind of sugar called gentianose, which occurs only in the gentian family of plants; an abundance of fat oil; mineral salts.

MEDICINAL USE: The root—*Radix Gentianae*.

A decoction of the gentian root has long been used externally by mountain dwellers as a strengthening foot-bath and as a poultice on badly healing or suppurating wounds.

More important, however, is its internal use. In cases of heartburn, indigestion, loss of appetite, nausea and sluggish bowel movement, the tea made from 2–3 grams (30.8–46.2 grains avdp) boiled 5 minutes in 2 cups of water, if drunk before meals, has a stimulating effect on the entire range of metabolic processes. Gout and rheumatism are also beneficially influenced. The tea is recommended by physicians for all conditions of weakness. Gentian root is *not* used to counter excessive inflammation, tendency toward excitement, passive (or venous) hyperaemia (excess blood in a part of the body), or hemorrhages. People with a tendency toward headache should avoid gentian.

CULINARY USE: Gentiane, a highly prized digestive liqueur, is distilled from the yellow gentian in France and Switzerland.

GERMANDER

SCIENTIFIC NAME: *Teucrium scorodonia.*

OTHER POPULAR NAMES: Wood sage, wood germander, wood sage germander.

FAMILY: Labiatae—Mint Family.

RANGE: Germander thrives in western Europe in stony soil and along the edges of woods, in forest glades and felled clearings. There are two closely related North American forms—*T. canadense* and *T. occidentale.*

DESCRIPTION: The stem climbs slim and tall from the root, laden with opposed, oval, sharp-pointed leaves that are hairy and dull green. From the upper leaf axes, slim spikes also climb toward the light, bearing pale-yellowish, labiate flowers.

ELEMENTS CONTAINED: Essential oil, a bitter principle, silicic acid.

MEDICINAL USE: The plant—*Herba Teucrii.*

Used externally in folk medicine for faster healing and cicatrizing (scab-forming) of wounds. The tea made from 15–20 grams ($\frac{1}{2}-\frac{2}{3}$ ounce) of the whole plant, is used as an inhalant, the vapors being inhaled in cases of mouth and throat troubles as well as sinus catarrh.

The greatest effect of the plant when taken internally is known to be in cases of tuberculosis of the lungs, bones, joints and glands.

CULINARY USE: None.

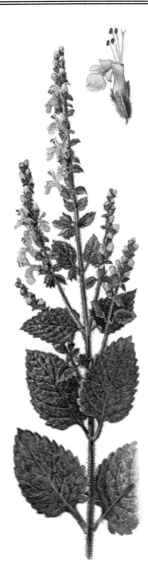

Germander

GROMWELL

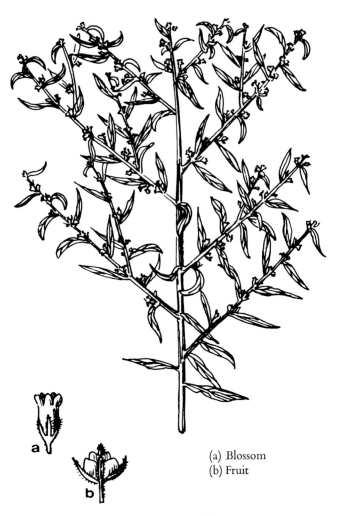

SCIENTIFIC NAME: *Lithospermum officinale.*
OTHER POPULAR NAME: Common gromwell.
FAMILY: Boraginaceae—Borage Family.
RANGE: In Europe, this plant grows in sandy-stony places, as it is mostly found in river valleys and many times in fields. It is widely naturalized in the eastern United States.
DESCRIPTION: Lanceolate leaves stand on a branched stalk. From the axes of the leaves grow inconspicuous, little white blossoms, which bloom in early summer. In late summer, many fruits emerge from the flowers by fours, gleaming like pearls.
ELEMENTS CONTAINED: Gromwell is the herb which is richest in silicic acid. It also contains tannic acids, fat oil, and lime.
MEDICINAL USE: Seeds—*Semen Lithospermi.*

The leaves of this plant are rich in tannin and used to be used in teas. The seeds, which are very rich in lime and silicic acid, are diuretic and have a beneficial effect on kidney conditions. Take 1–4 grams (15.4–61.6 grains avdp) of the drug and boil in 1 cup of water. After steeping, strain. In America, a similar species, *Lithospermum ruderale*, has long been taken by Indian tribes as an agent for preventing conception. The native European gromwell also appears to have this effect, which derives from plant hormones, but no such use has yet been developed.
CULINARY USE: None.

(a) Blossom
(b) Fruit

Gromwell

GROUND IVY

SCIENTIFIC NAMES: *Glechoma hederacea, Nepeta glechoma, Nepeta hederacea.*

OTHER POPULAR NAMES: Gill, ale-hoof, haymaids, gill-over-the-ground, gill-go-by-the-ground, field-balm, cats' foot, turn-hoof.

FAMILY: Labiatae—Mint Family.

RANGE: Along fences, hedges, roads and on walls and wet meadows throughout central Europe. Also common in the United States, growing in shady places, waste grounds, dry ditches, etc.

DESCRIPTION: Ground ivy is one of the first plants to show itself in the spring. From its creeping, ever self-renewing runners, it sends up inflorescences with blue-violet, labiate flowers. The roundish, notched leaves are set in pairs on the vertical stem, and the flowers grow from their axes.

ELEMENTS CONTAINED: A bitter principle, choline, tannin, essential oil, gummy substances, mineral substances, salts.

MEDICINAL USE: The whole plant when in flower—*Herba Hederae terrestris.*

Ground ivy is used externally for poultices in a decoction of 10 grams (154 grains avdp) in $\frac{1}{2}$ litre (1 pint) of water. Pour boiling water over a handful of this plant to use as an herbal addition to a bath. Such baths heal aging, badly healing wounds and assuage the pain of neuralgia, sciatica, gout and toothache.

For internal use, take either the tincture or a decoction—5–10 grams (77–154 grains avdp) in $\frac{1}{2}$ litre (1 pint) of water. Use the plant internally and externally for regulating the metabolism in spleen-liver congestion, weakness of the digestive tract, deficiency in blood building, in cases of bronchial asthma, disease of the breathing organs, scrofula, stone and yellow jaundice.

CULINARY USE: The closely related catnip or catmint *(Nepeta cataria)* is used to make an herbal tea, and the dried leaves, as is well known, are a treat for cats. Before the introduction of hops into England (16th century) ground ivy was used to give beer a sharper taste.

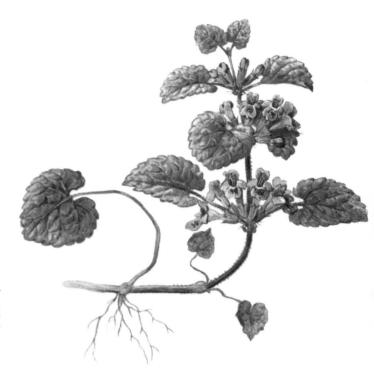

Ground Ivy

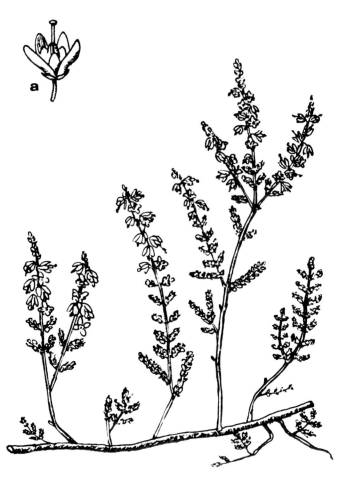

(a) Blossom

Heather

HEATHER

SCIENTIFIC NAMES: *Calluna vulgaris, Erica vulgaris.*
OTHER POPULAR NAMES: Common heath, ling.
FAMILY: Ericaceae—Heath Family.
RANGE: Heather knows how to defy the sun and by thick growth to retain the slightest existing moisture in the soil. This plant is found in lime-poor soil on the heaths of Europe and Britain, in bogs, on sand dunes and in forest glades, and has spread to Greenland and parts of North America. It grows in high northern latitudes, and in mountains up to an altitude of 2,000 m (6,600 ft).
DESCRIPTION: This low, dwarf bush covers poor soil in large stands. The woody, decumbent stem with its out-thrusting branches develops thick bushes 10–50 cm (4–20 inches) high, bearing evergreen, needle-shaped leaflets. The numerous ends of the erected sprouts bear clusters of small reddish-violet (many times also white) blossoms, which cover broad moors and upland meadows from July into September with a purple carpet and offer the bees a rich feast.
ELEMENTS CONTAINED: Flavone glycosides, tannin, saponin, sugar, gum, and mineral substances, including plentiful lime and silicic acid.
MEDICINAL USE: The blooming plant—*Herba Ericae cum floribus.* Blossoms—*Flores Ericae.*

On account of its diuretic effect, heather is used in cases of gout, rheumatism, kidney and gall-stone complaints. In this way, it also relieves the heart and circulatory system. For the tea, 2–4 grams (30.8–61.6 grains avdp) of the plant or the flowers are scalded in 1 cup of boiling water.
CULINARY USE: Heather is often an ingredient of breakfast and domestic tea.

POISON HEMLOCK

SCIENTIFIC NAME: *Conium maculatum.*

OTHER POPULAR NAMES: Hemlock, cowbane, spotted hemlock, common hemlock, poison root, cicuta, spotted cowbane, poison snakeweed.

FAMILY: Umbelliferae—Parsley or Carrot Family.

RANGE: In Europe and northern Asia, poison hemlock grows everywhere along river banks and streams and on the shores of ponds, and has also been naturalized in North and South America.

DESCRIPTION: Of the 2,200 species of hemlock, only a few are tropical and none are trees. The unrelated North American hemlock tree is a conifer of the genus *Tsuga* of the Pine Family. The poison hemlock grows to a height of 2 metres (80 inches). In the first year of growth, the plant forms a spindle-shaped root and the lower leaves and develops a whitish, milky sap. The following year, a hollow, purple-spotted stem shoots up. The leaves are triply and quadruply pinnate (that is, each leaf is divided into leaflets which in turn are divided and redivided, each leaflet appearing to be a tiny separate leaf) and exhibit a whitish border around their edges. On hot summer days, the entire foliage hangs slack and shrivelled, because the abundantly articulated, delicate leaves quickly evaporate their water into the air, faster than fresh water can climb up from the ground. The umbels end in slightly sweetish-scented, white umbellets. A cloud of scent more suggestive of animals than plants surrounds the entire herb.

ELEMENTS CONTAINED: The alkaloid conine (coniine) is present in the root up to 0.05 per cent, in the stem up to 0.06 per cent, in the leaves up to 0.02 per cent, and in the flowers up to 0.24 per cent. An intake of 0.15–0.2 gram ($1\frac{1}{2}$–3 grains) is fatal.

MEDICINAL USE: The plant—*Herba Conii.*

Even in ancient times, hemlock was known not only as a poison, but also as a medicinal plant. (Socrates killed himself with a dose of hemlock.) In the Middle Ages, too, the healing power of this plant was valued. Unfortunately, many of their experiments miscarried.

Today, hemlock is prescribed for external use as an anodyne (pain-assuaging), inflammation-restraining, emollient and resolving agent. Applied to glands, it hampers their function. Thus milk flow is affected and enlargement of the breasts prevented.

Internal doses increase secretion, drain off water and have a

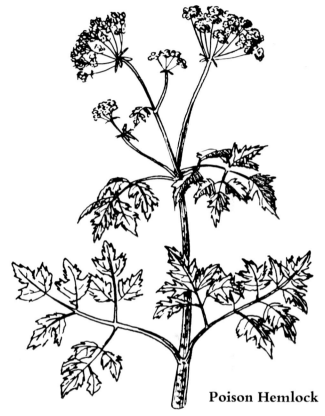

Poison Hemlock

(See illustration, page 122)

tranquilizing effect. In cases of hemlock poisoning, consciousness and heart action are maintained to the end. States of nervous excitement and mental confusion hardly ever appear. Hemlock is also an antispasmodic and for this reason is effective in cases of whooping cough, asthma, cramps in the digestive tract and the bladder, and in epilepsy. Use should be undertaken only under direct supervision of a physician.

CULINARY USE: None. Poisonous.

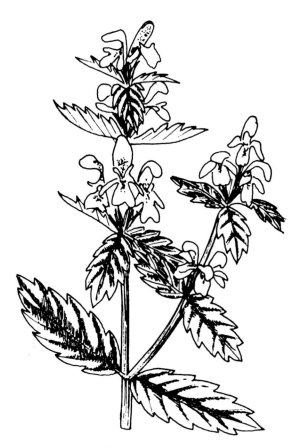

Hemp Nettle

HEMP NETTLE

SCIENTIFIC NAME: *Galeopsis segetum.*

OTHER POPULAR NAME: Dead nettle.

FAMILY: Labiatae—Mint Family.

RANGE: This plant is widespread in western Europe and prefers gravelly, sandy rubble-soil which, however, must be well wetted throughout. The closely related *G. tetrahit* of Europe and Asia has become a widespread weed in North America.

DESCRIPTION: This hemp-like plant with outspread, tooth-edged leaves and large, bright yellow, labiate flowers occurs in other varieties, one that blooms purple-red, one bright purple with a yellow and red flecked underlip, and the golden-yellow blooming hemp nettle with a violet spot. Common to all are the tooth-like, hollow protrusions of the lower jaw of the blossom, which give it the look of a widespread maw of an animal, which explains the Greek name *Galeopsis* (weasel face).

ELEMENTS CONTAINED: 3–10 per cent mineral substances, of which $\frac{1}{5}$ to $\frac{1}{3}$ is salicic acid; in addition, tannin, pectin, sugar, and saponin.

MEDICINAL USE: The whole plant when in bloom—*Herba Galeopsidis.*

Hemp nettle is a mild, diuretic remedy which has a beneficial effect on diseases of the lungs. On account of its high content of mineral substances, it is recommended for anemia. For internal use, pour 1 cup of boiling water over 1 tablespoonful of the plant.

CULINARY USE: None.

HORSE-RADISH

SCIENTIFIC NAMES: *Armoracia rusticana (Cochlearia armoracia, Radicula armoracia).*

OTHER POPULAR NAMES: None.

FAMILY: Cruciferae—Mustard Family.

RANGE: The horse-radish is native to southeast Europe, occasionally found growing wild, and cultivated in some parts of Europe. The plant runs wild in the United States, as well as being cultivated as an annual crop. Horse-radish does not propagate by seed but by root cuttings.

DESCRIPTION: The horse-radish plant is mainly root. The long-lived, main root reaches deep into the earth and sends far-reaching runners out in all directions. In addition, it forms suckers or shoots. Wherever these roots have once gained a foothold, they are very difficult ever to root out again. Coarse, lush green leaves 1 metre (40 inches) long are sent upward. They have a wavy shape, with notched edges, and take a spiral turn. The flower shoot bears loose clusters of white blossoms that have a sweet scent. The tiny little pods are thick and almost round.

ELEMENTS CONTAINED: The whole plant, but especially the root, contains the glycoside sinigrin (potassium myronate), which yields mustard oil after the root has been chopped fine and the enzyme myrosin that is present has been washed out with water. Ashes of the leaves show a high potash and sulphur content, as well as silicic acid. In the root ashes, some iron accompanies the above substances.

MEDICINAL USE: The root—*Radix Armoraciae.*

Horse-radish is highly valued for its influence on the skin as a counter-irritant. By means of baths, salves, and poultices (horse-radish plaster), with rubbed-in horse-radish, the pains of neuralgia, sciatica, cramps, pleurisy, joint and muscular rheumatism are beneficially influenced, as well as gout.

CULINARY USE: It has a very sharp and burning aroma and taste. The sharpness is mitigated by boiling. Fresh: Grated root. Dried: Powder before use, stir into plenty of water and let steep for $\frac{1}{2}$ hour.

Whip into sauces with cream, butter, mayonnaise, or grated apple, as a supplement to beef, sausage, ham, liver paste, fish, and similar dishes.

After grating, sprinkling with lemon prevents discoloring.

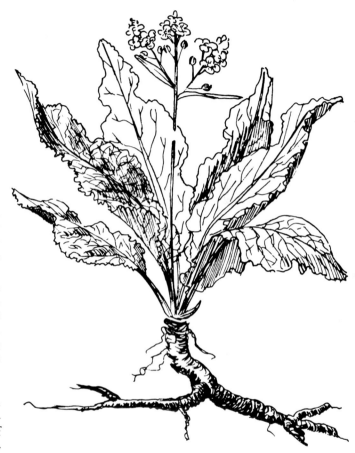

Horse-radish

Horsetail

SCIENTIFIC NAME: *Equisetum arvense.*

OTHER POPULAR NAMES: Horsetail grass, pewter grass, shave grass, cat's tail, field horsetail, field cat's tail, field equisetum, paddock pipes.

FAMILY: Equisetaceae—Horsetail Family (the only genus).

RANGE: Spread over almost the entire northern hemisphere, horsetail can usually be found on dry ground and in fields.

DESCRIPTION: Horsetails are among the earliest plants on earth. In the remote past, horsetails grew to an impressive size and, along with ferns and lycopodium (club-moss), formed gigantic forests in the then warm, humid climate of what are now temperate latitudes. Today, only a few large stands of giant horsetails are found; in the Amazon region, they are about 6 m (20 feet) high, while the tallest European species reach a height of 2 m (about $6\frac{1}{2}$ feet). The *Equisetum arvense* is only a modest little plant, whose root-stock (rhizome) is shaped like a string of beads. In the spring it sends up a 10-20-cm-high (4-8-inch) stalk of a straw-yellow hue. At intervals of 2-3 cm ($\frac{3}{4}$-$1\frac{1}{4}$ inches) the stalk bears ring-shaped leaf sheathes with many sharp little teeth. At the top, the stalk bears a club-shaped spike. This stalk bears the spores—for horsetail, like ferns, does not reproduce by seed. When the spore-bearing stalk dies away, the mature plant, of very different appearance, replaces it—a green plant with equally-spaced whorls of 10-12 branches.

ELEMENTS CONTAINED: Silicic acid, a bitter principle, oxalic acid, malic acid, peptohydrochloric acid, lime, sodium and potassium salts, iron, sulphur, manganese, magnesium, resin.

MEDICINAL USE: The sterile (mature) stalk and the branches are the parts used, called, in pharmacy, *Herba Equiseti.* For external use, horsetail tea is made by pouring 1 cup of boiling water over 1 to 4 grams (= 1 teaspoonful to 1 heaping tablespoonful) and is used for packs, baths, enemas, cleansing, washing, and as a gargle, in cases of festering wounds, leg sores, fistulas (including rectal), eczema, boils, inflammation of the eyelid, styes, proud-flesh in wounds, caries, and softening of the gums.

Internally, horsetail tea has a beneficial effect on bladder complaints, pulmonary disease, urinary calculus (gravel) and stones, dropsy, hemorrhages, and rheumatism.

CULINARY USE: None.

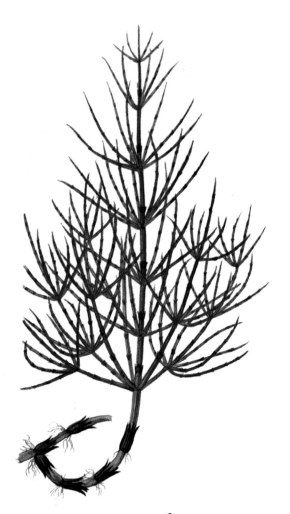

Horsetail

IRIS

SCIENTIFIC NAMES: *Iris germanica (Iris vulgaris).*
OTHER POPULAR NAMES: Flag iris, German iris.
FAMILY: Iridaceae—Iris Family.
RANGE: *Iris germanica* grows wild in the northern temperate zone, but it is mostly found in gardens. It is the ancestor of the cultivated, tall, bearded iris.
DESCRIPTION: From the 5–12-cm- (2–4¾-inch-) long, bulbous, articulated root, a powerful stem shoots upward, set around with long, sword-shaped leaves. A large, distinctive, violet flower with a three-part everted calyx and 3 petal-like appendages surrounding the stigma, crowns the tip.
ELEMENTS CONTAINED: Myristin (fat), oleic acid, irrone (the violet scent component), tannic acid, resin, methyl ether, a glycoside, iridin.
MEDICINAL USE: The root (violet-root)—*Rhizoma Iridis*; violet-root powder—*Rhizoma Iridis pulveratus*; peeled violet-root—*Radix Iridis mundatus.*

Violet-root was formerly used externally, sprinkled on unclean wounds to cleanse them. Small, rounded pieces are given to teething children to chew on.

Internal doses (1 tablespoonful of the finely chopped root boiled in 1 cup of water) are given in cases of spleen and gall-bladder disease and for mucous obstruction of the chest. It is also used as a diuretic.
CULINARY USE: None.

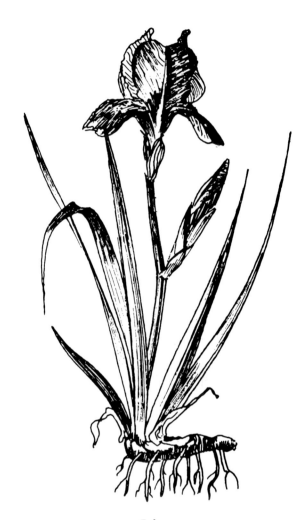

Iris

KNOTWEED

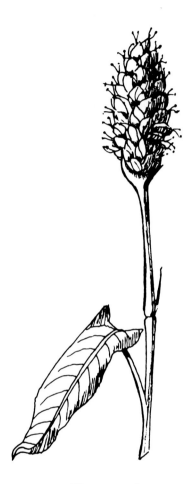

Knotweed

SCIENTIFIC NAME: *Polygonum bistorta*.

OTHER POPULAR NAMES: Fleece flower, snakeweed, bistort, snake-root, adder's-wort, patience dock, dragon weed.

FAMILY: Polygonaceae—Buckwheat or Knotweed Family.

RANGE: In Europe, knotweed occurs along ditches and on damp mountain meadows, where it often overruns other plants and looks as if it had been sowed. A similar plant, *P. bistortoides*, is found in North America.

DESCRIPTION: The most striking thing about this plant is the snake-like, twisted, curled, finger-thick (older plants are thumb-thick) root that is brown on the outside and which the knotweed has to thank for its name. Out of this root-stock, which has a great many secondary roots, comes an unbranched, knotty stem with sorrel-like leaves, crowned by a beautiful, pink, erect blossom spike.

ELEMENTS CONTAINED: Tannin and starch.

MEDICINAL USE: The root-stock—*Rhizoma Bistortae*.

In folk medicine, knotweed used to be used against various kinds of bleeding and, in many places, against snakebite. Up to now, modern medicine has been unable to recognize any visible medicinal value and for this reason does not use the plant for therapeutic purposes. In old-time herbals, it is often mentioned to the contrary.

CULINARY USE: In former times, bistort was used in England as a pot-herb, and was the chief ingredient of an Easter pudding traditionally served in the northern part of the country.

LADY'S MANTLE

SCIENTIFIC NAME: *Alchemilla vulgaris.*

OTHER POPULAR NAMES: Common lady's mantle, common alchemil.

FAMILY: Rosaceae—Rose Family.

RANGE: Lady's mantle grows throughout central Europe on meadows and along the edges of fields and woods, as well as on slopes and ridges. It has been naturalized in parts of eastern Canada. A closely related European species, *A. arvensis*, has been naturalized over much of the United States.

DESCRIPTION: Leaves sprout from the root-stock on long stems, rather like umbrellas twisted in a storm, appearing first folded together, then opening out into a convex surface. The leaves have the property of secreting water droplets in the morning and thereby take over what amounts practically to a flower function. These silver droplets collect on tiny hairs on the surface of the leaf. Alchemists used to gather the drops, as they thought that this "heavenly water" would aid them in preparing the Philosopher's Stone. That is how the plant received its Latin name of *alchemilla*. The inflorescence exhibits a very scanty arrangement of greenish blossoms, though their honey-sweet scent betrays their floral nature.

ELEMENTS CONTAINED: Tannin, a bitter principle, saponin.

MEDICINAL USE: The plant—*Herba Alchemillae.*

Lady's mantle is a real help in childbirth. A tea is made of 2–4 grams (30.8–61.6 grains avdp) of the plant scalded in 1 cup boiling water. Let steep 5 minutes, then strain. This is given following childbirth to promote healing of wounds and the stanching of blood. The plant also has a beneficial influence on menstrual disorders.

CULINARY USE: None.

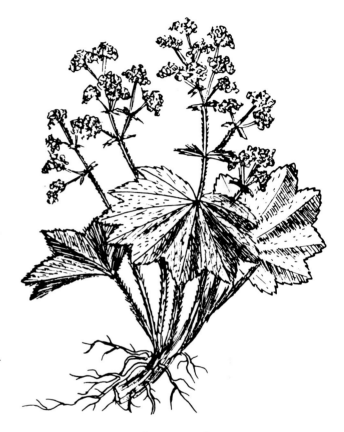

Lady's Mantle

FIELD LARKSPUR

SCIENTIFIC NAME: *Delphinium consolida.*
OTHER POPULAR NAMES: Forking larkspur, lark heel, knight's spur.
FAMILY: Ranunculaceae—Crowfoot or Buttercup Family.
RANGE: Field larkspur has spread practically all over Europe, yet it is rare in many districts. It grows in or near grain fields.
DESCRIPTION: The field larkspur belongs to a subdivision of the Crowfoot Family, the Hellebores, which are distinguished from other subdivisions of this family by the inward dehiscence (bursting open of the pod or capsule) of the encapsulated fruit. This beautiful field flower has an irregular flower structure, differing from the typical members of the buttercup tribe, for the uppermost of the 5 dissimilar, blue calyx leaves is lengthened into a spur, which makes the bud similar to that of a garden delphinium.
ELEMENTS CONTAINED: A bitter principle, tannin, dyestuff.
MEDICINAL USE: The blossoms—*Flores Calcatrippae.*

In the Middle Ages, physicians considered this plant an outstanding healing agent for wounds, as it was supposed to close the wound quickly and cause it to heal. An infusion made from 2–4 grams (30.8–61.6 grains avdp) scalded with 1 cup of boiling water, used to serve as a diuretic and a worming agent. Also, larkspur was valued as a remedy for healing sore eyes. Yet, up to now, modern medicine has found no special healing effect, for which reason this plant is very little used today in medicine.

Today, the blossoms are used only as a side-ingredient in tea mixtures to give the tea coloration. The seeds are said to have a good effect on spasmodic coughing.
CULINARY USE: None.

Field Larkspur

Lavender

SCIENTIFIC NAME: *Lavandula officinalis (L. spica* and *L. vera).*
OTHER POPULAR NAMES: Spikenard, nard, spike lavender.
FAMILY: Labiatae—Mint Family.
RANGE: The sunny, dry slopes of the western Mediterranean, the Canary Islands and India are the native habitat of this light- and warmth-loving plant. Elsewhere it is planted in gardens and parks.
DESCRIPTION: Climbing upward from the ground, the sprout branches out and creates a low bush with soft, needle-like, bluish-green leaves out of which the flower spikes broadly project in a soft, pure, lavender-blue, suffusing the air of the mountain slopes with their perfume.
ELEMENTS CONTAINED: Lavender contains in its dried blossoms 1.5–3 per cent essential oil, of which the most important constituent is linalool. In addition, both geraniol and cumarin are present. Other constituents are resin, tannin, and a bitter principle.
MEDICINAL USE: The flowers—*Flores Lavandulae*; oil—*Oleum Lavandulae.*

Lavender stimulates the activity of the metabolism and is thereby soothing, calming, antispasmodic, sleep-inducing, and nerve-strengthening. For tea, 2 grams (30.8 grains avdp) of the dried blossoms are scalded with 1 cup of boiling water. Kneipp recommended 5 drops of lavender oil twice a day for headaches, flatulency, loss of appetite, and for stimulation of the digestion. As a bath additive, lavender helps in cases of rheumatism, gout, and sciatica.

CULINARY USE: Lavender is used rarely as a seasoning similar to rosemary. However, dried lavender (usually in packets) is used in keeping clothes closets sweet smelling.

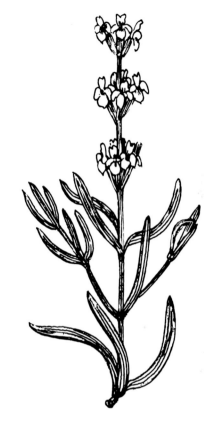

Lavender

LEEK

SCIENTIFIC NAME: *Allium porrum*.

OTHER POPULAR NAME: Wild leek.

FAMILY: Liliaceae—Lily Family.

RANGE: Believed to have originated in Asia, the leek came to Europe at an early date (it is the national emblem of Wales) and has been naturalized sparingly in North America. A North American species, the wild leek *(A. tricoccum)*, is a common woodland plant.

DESCRIPTION: The leek is a hardy biennial herb of the onion genus. It is characterized by broad leaves 2 inches (5 cm) wide and 2–3 feet (60–90 cm) long, which overlap toward their base, forming a sort of bundle. The small pink flowers form dense, rounded terminal clusters. The whole plant has a smell of onions, but milder than the onion itself.

ELEMENTS CONTAINED: Proteins, vitamin C, essential oil, sulphur.

MEDICINAL USE: As a diuretic and blood-building agent.

CULINARY USE: The leek, along with fowl, is a main ingredient of the Scottish national dish, cock-a-leekie. The whole plant, except for the small fibrous roots, is added to stews, ragouts, soups such as Scotch broth, braised beef and other dishes. Leeks are one of the indispensable items of French cookery, especially in the preparation of soups—the standard soup in homes and restaurants alike is based on leeks and potatoes.

Leek

Prickly Lettuce

SCIENTIFIC NAME: *Lactuca virosa*.

OTHER POPULAR NAMES: Poison lettuce, acrid lettuce, lettuce opium, lettuce.

FAMILY: Compositae—Composite Family.

RANGE: Prickly lettuce, close kin to the wholesome garden lettuce, is found on fallow land, stony slopes, and along the edges of fields in Europe, North Africa and in western Asia. It has been naturalized in parts of North America, where it has become a troublesome weed. A similar species, *L. saligna*, is found in Australia.

DESCRIPTION: This plant was formerly used along with henbane and hemlock as a narcotic in surgery. It is a biennial and in its first year develops a sturdy taproot and a rosette of dandelion-like leaves. When the hollow stem in the following year reaches a height of 1 metre (40 inches), the amplexicaul, blue-green leaves divide. The leaf-veins show thorn-like growths on their undersides. The ends of the stems develop many-flowered panicles, with the composite flowers forming yellow heads. From these, in the autumn, feathery little parachutes carry the seeds off into the distance. The entire plant is gorged with milky sap.

ELEMENTS CONTAINED: Lactucarium (lettuce opium) is obtained by air-drying the milky sap. This contains a crystallizable, nitrogen-free bitter principle (lactucopicrin and lactucin), traces of an alkaloid, asparagine, organic acids, camphor, mannite, rubber (caoutchouc), and some essential oil.

MEDICINAL USE: The plant in bloom—*Herba Lactucae virosae*.

Prickly lettuce has sedative, cough preventative, and antispasmodic effects; however, it does not assuage pain nor clear phlegm. This medicinal plant beneficially affects enlargement of the liver and cramps in the region of the bladder and bowels. It suppresses nervous conditions, and, thanks to its properties, it saves using opiates and does not cause addiction.

CULINARY USE: Although prickly lettuce is classified as narcotic and poisonous, the very young leaves, picked when the plant is only a few inches high, are used by some people as a salad and pot-herb.

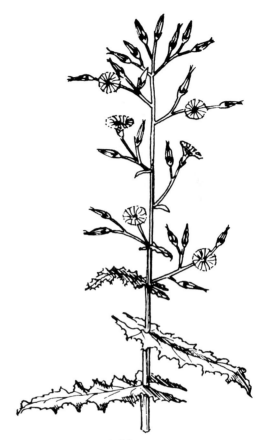

Prickly Lettuce

Lily-of-the-Valley

LILY-OF-THE-VALLEY

SCIENTIFIC NAME; *Convallaria majalis*.

OTHER POPULAR NAMES: May lily, May blossom, park lily.

FAMILY: Liliaceae—Lily Family.

RANGE: The comely little bell-like flower blooms in the moderately wet half-shade of cool, deciduous forests, early foreshadowing the warmth of summer.

DESCRIPTION: Not until you have closely examined the appearance of this dainty little plant do you realize how fascinating it can be. In the autumn, the branched root-stock stops growing and produces nodules on its ends. From these in the spring two long-stemmed, elliptically pointed leaves appear out of the ground. Next, a leafless, erect flower-stalk comes up, surrounded by blossom nodes. When the white blossoms open, they turn themselves in the direction of the most light. Those on the other side also attempt to change their direction, but in doing so their weight causes the erect shaft to bend far over. Round, blood-red little fruits follow the little bell-like flowers; in these are concealed blue seeds. A world of contrasts exists in this little plant: It loves shade and yet seeks the light; it loves spring and grows on into the summer; its inflorescence strives straight upward and falls over from its own weight; the pure white of the blossoms is replaced by the bright red fruits, which contain blue seeds.

The scent of the lily-of-the-valley is sweet and cool, but when brought indoors soon causes a sensation of irritating pungency in the nostrils.

ELEMENTS CONTAINED: Essential oil and the poisons, convallarin and convallamarin.

MEDICINAL USE: Flowers and flower stems—*Flores Convallariae majalis*; leaves—*Folia Convallariae*.

Because it is poisonous, the lily-of-the-valley is not usable as a household remedy and its use and dosage must be left to the physician. As a medicinal plant, it exercises a healing influence on the beating heart, disturbances in the rhythm of the heart, especially in juveniles, raises the blood pressure, and relieves cramping in asthma.

CULINARY USE: None. Poisonous.

LIVERLEAF

SCIENTIFIC NAMES: *Hepatica nobilis, Anemone hepatica.*

OTHER POPULAR NAMES: Hepatica, liverwort, crystalwort. (Kidney liverleaf, for *Hepatica americana*.)

FAMILY: Ranunculaceae—Crowfoot or Buttercup Family.

RANGE: The liverleaf grows throughout Europe in shady woods. American species include *Hepatica americana* and *H. acutaloba*, which have the same medicinal effect. *Hepatica nobilis* is confined to continental Europe.

DESCRIPTION: When in the spring the first rays of the sun have melted the snow, this tender little flower pops up unexpectedly. Its pure, blue blossoms withstand the cold of frost and snow. Entire blue carpets cover the forest floor and the brown leaves of the previous year. The beautiful flower has well shaped, triple-lobed petals, softly haired. The 7-petalled, round blossom is pure blue.

ELEMENTS CONTAINED: The plant contains a volatile, nitrogen-free compound, anemon, which, on drying the plant, divides into the constituents anemonin, anemon, and isoanemonic acid. Anemonol is a topical and very irritating poison, which upon resorption leads first to stimulation and then to paralysis of the central nervous system. This poison completely disappears upon drying the plant. In addition, the following are also present: tannin, resin, a glycoside (hypatrilolin), and saponin in the root-stock.

MEDICINAL USE: The plant—*Herba Hepaticae nobilis.*

The dried plant is given as an astringent and powerful remedy principally in liver and gall troubles. The solution is made from 2–4 grams (30.8–61.6 grains avdp) of the dried plant, scalded with 1 cup of boiling water.

CULINARY USE: None.

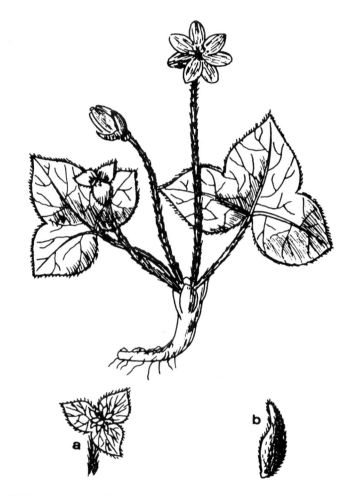

(a) Fruit-bearing calyx
(b) Single fruit (enlarged)

Liverleaf

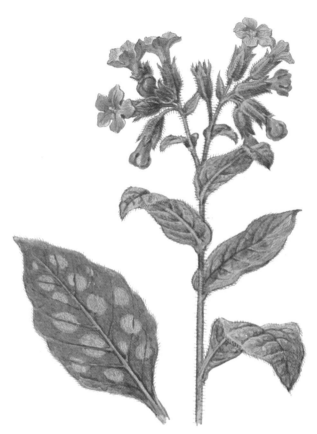

Lungwort

LUNGWORT

SCIENTIFIC NAMES: *Pulmonaria officinalis (P. maculata).*
OTHER POPULAR NAMES: Sage of Bethlehem, maple lungwort.
FAMILY: Boraginaceae—Borage Family.
RANGE: This plant is tolerably widespread in the greater part of Europe, from Sweden as far south as the northern Balkans, and in north and central Italy, and is also found in many parts of North America. It grows mainly in light, not too dry, deciduous forests. It is also suitable for the flower garden and border.
DESCRIPTION: When the light of spring still penetrates unhindered to the ground through the leafless crowns of the trees, the lungwort grows from a horizontally creeping root. Its alternating leaves seem to respond to the play of light and shadow with white flecks. Its flowers have a great similarity to those of the cowslip, their shades changing, however, from a bright reddish-violet upon blooming to blue.
ELEMENTS CONTAINED: Mucilage, tannin, fat, resin, phlobaphene, invert sugar (mixture of equal molecules of dextrose and levulose), polysaccharides, mineral substances, silicic acid, saponin.
MEDICINAL USE: The plant—*Herba Pulmonariae.*

Lungwort is used externally for the healing of wounds. A decoction is made from the powdered root and lower leaves and applied to the affected area. The powder is also sprinkled around the edges of the wound and over the inflamed area.

Internally, a tea is given of 2 grams (30.8 grains avdp) of the plant, scalded in 1 cup of boiling water. At regular intervals throughout the day, the patient drinks a total of 3 cups of tea for lung disease (even for tuberculosis of the lungs), hemoptysis (hemorrhage from larynx, trachea or lungs), bronchitis, inflammation of the throat, and hoarseness, as well as for hematuria (blood in the urine), bladder weakness, dysentery, and diarrhea.
CULINARY USE: None.

Lycopodium

SCIENTIFIC NAME: *Lycopodium clavatum*.

OTHER POPULAR NAMES: Club moss, ground pine, ground fir, running pine, common club moss, witch meal, vegetable sulphur, staghorn moss.

FAMILY: Lycopodiaceae—Club Moss Family.

RANGE: Lycopodium occurs on dry heaths, on mountain slopes and in forests in Europe, North America and Asia. In Germany, the spore capsules (sporangia) are gathered in the Rhön mountains, in the Spessart highland forest district of Bavaria, and in the Harz Mountains.

DESCRIPTION: Lycopodium has a creeping stem bristling all round with tiny leaves. It grows to more than a metre (40 inches) long. Small twigs rise up along the creeping stem, on the tips of which stand long, thin, erect stalks, bearing on their ends two spike-like, yellowish-green sporangia (spore cases). There is a marked contrast between the long, horizontal stem, and the stiffly erect stems with their sporangia projecting into the air.

ELEMENTS CONTAINED: Analysis of the seed yields about 50 per cent fat oil, as well as sugar, acids, resin, and mucilage, and the ashes are rich in aluminium. The plant itself contains a bitter principle, fat, and resin.

MEDICINAL USE: The spores—*Sporae Lycopodii*; the whole plant—*Herba Lycopodii*. *Sporae Lycopodii* is used externally on the skin, especially in the form of a powder applied to counter soreness (excoriation) of the breast caused by suckling. Lycopodium powder adheres easily, is not soluble in water, and does not cake up.

Internally, the tea, 1–4 grams (15.4–61.6 grains avdp) scalded by pouring 1 cup of boiling water over it (or briefly boiled) is effective against bladder catarrh (cystitis) and bladder pains which appear in conjunction with catching cold. It is diuretic and purgative.

CULINARY USE: None.

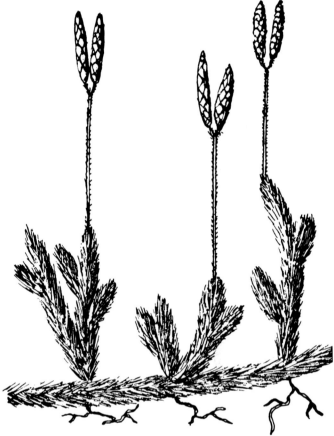

Lycopodium

MADDER

(a) Fruit   (b) Blossom

Madder

SCIENTIFIC NAME: *Rubia tinctorum*.

OTHER POPULAR NAMES: Dyer's cleavers, dyer's madders.

FAMILY: Rubiaceae—Madder Family.

RANGE: From ancient times to the 19th century, the plant was cultivated as an important source of red or rose-hued dye and paint, but is subject to fading. With the appearance of the synthetic, permanent dye, alizarin, madder disappeared from the fields. Since that time, it has grown wild.

DESCRIPTION: From a yard- (metre-) long, creeping root-stock rises a luxuriant plant with coarsely bristled leaves and stems whose shoots bear yellow-green blossoms, from which spring first red, then black, berries. The plant is similar in many ways to bedstraw.

ELEMENTS CONTAINED: Various kinds of sugar, pectin, a fat oil, citric acid, tannin, dye and a large quantity of minerals (a lot of potassium, 3.8 per cent sodium, a lot of lime, 6 per cent magnesium, 2.8 per cent iron, 9 per cent phosphoric acid, 3 per cent sulphuric acid, 16 per cent silicic acid, 13 per cent chlorine.)

MEDICINAL USE: The root—*Radix Rubiae tinctorum*.

Effective when used externally on skin ulcers, skin cancer, ulcers of the Adam's apple, and the mouth and throat. For this, 1–2 grams (15.4–30.8 grains avdp) of the root is boiled in 1 cup water, or is made into a cold decoction.

Internal use is particularly effective against kidney and bladder troubles. It combats the formation of stones, as well as inflammation and cramps. Madder turns the urine red and, with long use, the bones.

CULINARY USE: None.

MALLOW

SCIENTIFIC NAME: *Malva silvestris*.

OTHER POPULAR NAMES: Common mallow, wild mallow, common wild mallow, wild malva, high mallow, cheese flower.

FAMILY: Malvaceae—Mallow Family.

RANGE: Wild mallow grows all over the world along fences and roadsides, on rubbish and in quarries. It is naturalized in North America.

DESCRIPTION: The mallow plants form a family with an abundance of genera and species, among which, in the warm zones, are found shrubs such as the cotton plant, as well as mighty trees. The wild mallow proper *(Malva neglecta)* grows in central Europe, a decumbent species, along with the common mallow *(Malva silvestris)*. The last-named species grows to a height of a metre (about 40 inches), has a hairy stem, and 5- to 7-lobed, widely crenated leaves, from the axes of which grow small bouquets of pale, pinkish-red blossoms.

ELEMENTS CONTAINED: A great deal of mucilage, tannin, starch, a dyestuff (malvin).

MEDICINAL USE: The blossoms—*Flores Malvae silvestris*; the leaves —*Folia Malvae silvestris*.

For external use, a decoction (pour 1 cup of water over 1 teaspoonful of the plant and blossoms and boil briefly; let steep 5 minutes before straining) is made into an emollient poultice for hardened glands, ulcers and painful hemorrhoids. The decoction also helps in cases of inflammation of the throat and of mouth ulcers, when used as a gargle. Poultices for inflammation of the eyelids are equally recommendable.

Mallow tea is well known as a good remedy for internal use against bronchitis.

CULINARY USE: The leaves can be served uncooked in salads, or boiled like spinach.

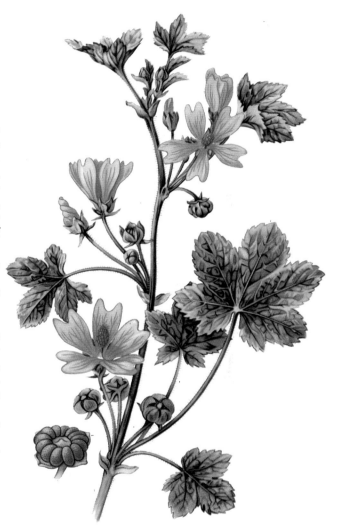

Mallow

Sweet Marjoram

Sweet Marjoram

SCIENTIFIC NAMES: *Origanum majorana (Majorana hortensis)*.

OTHER POPULAR NAMES: Garden marjoram, knotted marjoram, annual marjoram.

FAMILY: Labiatae—Mint Family.

RANGE: Native to the warm Mediterranean lands, this plant was valued by the ancient Greeks and Romans. It did not become widely known until the 16th century, and since then, it has been cultivated in gardens and nurseries.

DESCRIPTION: This charming plant has a life of two and sometimes more years. On its branched stalks, it forms short-stemmed, roundish leaves and flower spikes, with little white labiate blossoms almost covered with round, glandular bracteoles.

ELEMENTS CONTAINED: Essential oil, camphor-like substances, fat oil, tannin.

MEDICINAL USE: The plant—*Herba Majoranae*.

This beloved kitchen herb strengthens stomach and intestines, helps in cases of colic, flatulency and diarrhea as well as by reason of its antispasmodic character in cases of asthma, paralyzation, and attacks of giddiness. In preparation of a tea, take 2–4 grams (1–2 tablespoonfuls) of the plant and pour over it 1 cup of boiling water.

Just before the Second World War, marjoram salve was a valued and respected remedy for nasal blockage, catarrh, especially in children on account of its mild effect, and was rubbed in to resolve caked breast.

CULINARY USES: Very spicy aroma, lingering taste. Used fresh: Chop the leaves fine. Dried: Rubbed or ground. Use with meat, game, poultry, soups, gravies, stews, vegetables, and in the preparation of sausage.

Chopped green on bread and butter, bread spread with curds, and on greens. Greens should not be boiled. Keep dried marjoram in an airtight container. Green marjoram can also be frozen.

MARSHMALLOW

SCIENTIFIC NAME: *Althaea officinalis.*

OTHER POPULAR NAMES: Sweet weed, wymote, althaea, marsh althaea, guimauve.

FAMILY: Malvaceae—Mallow Family.

RANGE: In Europe, the marshmallow grows in soils containing salt—along the seashore, in wet meadows and by rivers and inland lakes which have a small salt content. In many regions, marshmallow is cultivated, especially in the Franconia region of Germany.

DESCRIPTION: From the fleshy root climbs an erect, felt-like stem whose broadly oval, tooth-edged and weakly trilobate leaves are overlaid with a soft, silky down. The flowers are pink, their anthers violet.

ELEMENTS CONTAINED: Mucilage, sugar, fat oil, some essential oil, starch, pectin, phytosterol, asparagine, lecithin, enzymes, tannin, malic acid, phosphorus.

MEDICINAL USE: Marshmallow flowers—*Flores Althaeae*; leaves—*Folia Althaeae*; root—*Radix Althaeae*.

Marshmallow is a remedy for coughs, hoarseness, bronchial and tracheal catarrh (bronchitis), and is not only highly recommended for adults but also for small children. In many commercially prepared mixtures of cough teas, marshmallow is found; it is also used in coughdrops and mouthwash. A home-made tea can be prepared from the blossoms, the leaves or the roots, by pouring a cup of boiling water over 2–5 grams (30.8–77 grains avdp) of the material. The roots (1 part to 10 parts water) are also suitable for preparation of a cold extract, which must be stirred often and left to soak for $1\frac{1}{2}$ hours.

Marshmallow tea also exercises a good effect on the digestive tract in cases of colic and even dysentery.

CULINARY USE: Used in Europe to make a confection in the form of a sweetened paste made from the root of the marshmallow. (TRANSLATOR'S NOTE: The United States confection in the form of white, sugared cubes called "marshmallows" is totally unrelated to the marshmallow. According to Webster, it is "a confection made of corn syrup, sugar, albumen, and gelatin, beaten to a light, creamy consistency and rolled in powdered sugar when partially dry.")

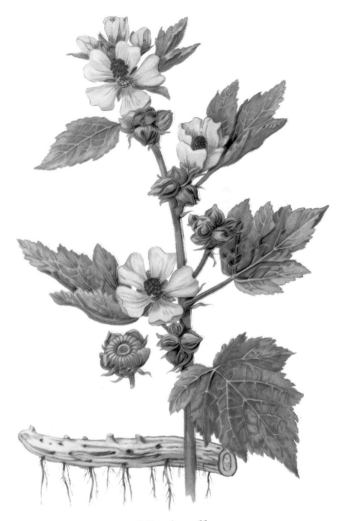

Marshmallow

MEADOWSWEET

SCIENTIFIC NAMES: *Filipendula ulmaria (F. pentapetala, Spiraea ulmaria)*.

OTHER POPULAR NAME: Queen-of-the-Meadow.

FAMILY: Rosaceae—Rose Family.

RANGE: This distinctive plant grows throughout Europe and in northern Asia on damp meadows, by ditches, swampy seashores, and among reeds along river courses. It is naturalized in eastern North America.

DESCRIPTION: The root-stock creeps through the wet, swampy ground, adding on a new piece each year, rooting from the nodes, and finally sends a shoot upward, which sprouts pinnate leaves, until the stately stem overflows at its tip in a white foam of blossom. The many-rayed false umbels of blossoms, whose hue is like yellowed linen, emanate a strong, bitter-sweet scent. The name meadowsweet is very apt, because the plants at haying time scent the meadows with their sweet smell.

ELEMENTS CONTAINED: Salicylic acid, a glycoside (gaultherin), essential oil, traces of heliotropin, vanillin.

MEDICINAL USE: The blossoms—*Flores Spiraeae ulmariae*; the root—*Radix Spiraeae ulmariae*.

Meadowsweet tea is made from 2–4 grams (30.8–61.6 grains avdp) scalded with 1 cup of boiling water and has a blood-purifying effect, is a diuretic and a diaphoretic, and for this reason is used for kidney and bladder troubles, dropsy, gout, and rheumatism with beneficial results.

CULINARY USE: None.

Meadowsweet

Yellow Melilot

SCIENTIFIC NAME: *Melilotus officinalis.*

OTHER POPULAR NAMES: Sweet clover, yellow sweet clover, melilot, common melilot.

FAMILY: Leguminosae—Pea or Pulse Family.

RANGE: Along roads and field borders, and on trash dumps, yellow melilot occurs everywhere in Europe, where the soil is rich in lime. It has been widely naturalized in the United States and Canada (it is also cultivated).

DESCRIPTION: This biennial plant drives its sturdy taproot deep into the ground and stands a metre (40 inches) high. The branched stalk exhibits long-stemmed, long, triple leaves having sharply saw-toothed edges. The small, yellow butterfly blossoms stand erect in long, loose clusters at the tips of the stems. The leaves as well as the flowers emit a honey-like fragrance.

ELEMENTS CONTAINED: Essential oil, melilotic acid, resin, cumarin, tannin and many salts.

MEDICINAL USE: The blossoms—*Flores Meliloti.* Plant in flower—*Herba Meliloti.*

Blossoms and plant are used externally as an emollient, pain-relieving, inflammation-retarding and resolving poultice in cases of swelling of joints or glands, ulcers, boils and wounds. For emollient poultices and washes, make up an infusion of 1 tablespoonful in $\frac{1}{2}$ litre (1 pint) of water.

Yellow melilot is hardly ever used internally, since over-use can cause vomiting and vertigo. It was often praised in old-time herbals on account of its soothing, sleep-promoting, diuretic and diaphoretic (sweat-inducing) effect. New scientific investigations have now revealed that yellow malilot has a tonic effect like horse-chestnut on the walls of the veins and therefore has the power of beneficial influence on varicose vein troubles.

CULINARY USE: None.

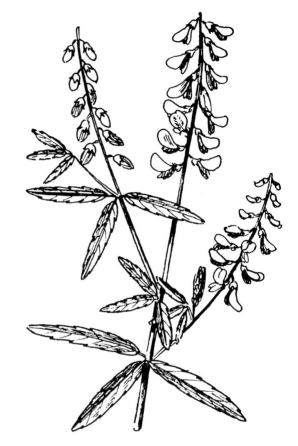

Yellow Melilot

Mezereon

SCIENTIFIC NAME: *Daphne mezereum.*

OTHER POPULAR NAMES: Paradise plant, magell, wild pepper, spurge flax, dwarf bay, spurge olive.

FAMILY: Thymelaceae—Mezereon Family.

RANGE: Mezereon grows throughout Eurasia up to the Arctic Circle, and has been naturalized in parts of North America.

DESCRIPTION: A few bare twigs left over from last year stand lost, stiff and stark among the trees. No one sees them, especially in the still wintry landscape. Yet, by March, there break forth from the twigs countless purplish-red flowers which emit an overpowering scent. The leaves do not come on until later and stand in clusters at the end of every twig. In the myths of the Germans and the Slavs, ribbons made from the *bast* (inner bark) can even overpower the devil.

ELEMENTS CONTAINED: A harsh, epispastic resin (tending to produce blisters), mezereonic acid, and a crystalline bitter principle called daphnin.

MEDICINAL USE: The bark—*Cortex Mezerei.*

Mezereon is used externally as a rub and as an ingredient in salves.

It is not often taken internally because of its harshness. How to use should be left to the physician.

CULINARY USE: None.

Mezereon

MILKWORT

SCIENTIFIC NAME: *Polygala amara* and any *Polygala* species, esp. *vulgaris*.

OTHER POPULAR NAMES: *Polygala vulgaris* is known also as: European senega, rogation flower, gang flower, common sea milkwort, and procession flower.

FAMILY: Polygalaceae—Milkwort Family.

RANGE: Milkwort prefers swampy, moor-like ground, or wet meadows, and thrives throughout Europe. *Polygala amara* and *vulgaris* are native to Europe, but other species of *Polygala* are native to North America.

DESCRIPTION: From a slender, fibrous root develops a rosette with oval leaves. Out of this climbs the flower-stem with leaves that are more spear-shaped, and a terminal cluster of dark blue blossoms. Less often, the blossoms are reddish or white.

ELEMENTS CONTAINED: Essential oil in traces, a crystalline bitter principle (polygalitol), wax, albumen, some fat oil, dyestuff, sugar, pectin, saponin, polygalic acid, mineral substances.

MEDICINAL USE: The plant—*Herba Polygalae amarae*.

Milkwort is used only internally. It was once thought to cause the flow of milk in nursing mothers, hence its name. As a result of its strong content of bitter principle, it is a superior remedy for stomach and intestinal troubles. Kneipp recommended it for bronchitis. It has proved itself in cases of lung disease, but should not be given, however, in cases of tuberculosis accompanied by fever or by bloody sputum. For tea, 1–3 grams (15.4–46.2 grains avdp) of the dried plant is scalded in 1 cup of boiling water.

CULINARY USE: None.

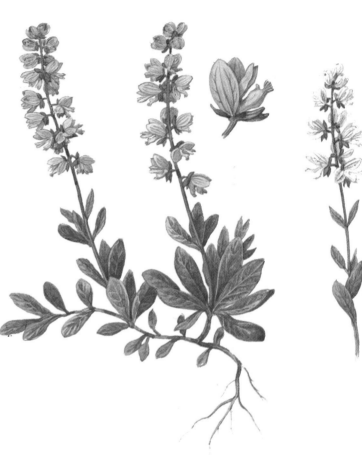

Milkwort

Mistletoe

SCIENTIFIC NAME: *Viscum album*.

OTHER POPULAR NAMES: Common mistletoe, white-berried mistletoe, bird lime, all-heal, devil's fuge.

FAMILY: Loranthaceae—Mistletoe Family.

RANGE: Mistletoe is known in northern Europe as a tree parasite and grows especially on the branches of deciduous trees. The mistletoe of literature is *Viscum album*, native from Great Britain to northern Asia. The mistletoe popular in North America at Christmas time is *Phoradendron flavescens* (originally *Viscum flavescens*), native from New Jersey to Florida and westward. *Viscum album* is confined to the Old World and Australia.

DESCRIPTION: Mistletoe is a peculiar plant. In winter, it decorates the leafless deciduous trees with its yellowish-green clusters, while its roots penetrate deep beneath the bark of its host in order to suck out its life-fluid. The green, articulated stems often fork and bear on the end two opposed, tongue-shaped, leathery leaves. In mid-winter, the blossoms sprout out of the last fork. The following winter, the mistletoe decks itself out with white, glistening berries and in England (and in America) is often present at Christmas celebrations. The fleshy fruit contains one seed, which often has several embryos, whose tiny roots already peep out of the seed. This has a connection with its unusual method of propagation. A large European thrush (mistle thrush or mistletoe thrush) swallows the berries and sows the embryos on the tree branches with its droppings.

ELEMENTS CONTAINED: Choline, an alkaloid, a resin-like bitter principle, a glycoside, an abundance of xanthophyll, a sticky, soft resin (viscin), glucose, inosite, starch, fat oil, an acidulous and a neutral saponin.

MEDICINAL USE: Plant—*Herba Visci* or *Stipites Visci cum foliis*.

The foremost importance of mistletoe is seen today in its influence through the blood pressure on the vegetative nervous system and hormone metabolism. Heart action and circulation are improved. Probably traceable to this characteristic is its use to combat bleedings of all kinds, such as lung bleeding, hematemesis (vomiting of blood from the stomach), and in cases of too heavy a menstrual flow (catamenia). Dosage: 3–6 grams (46.2–92.4 grains avdp) of the plant, scalded in 1 cup of boiling water.

CULINARY USE: None. However, traditionally lovers kiss without

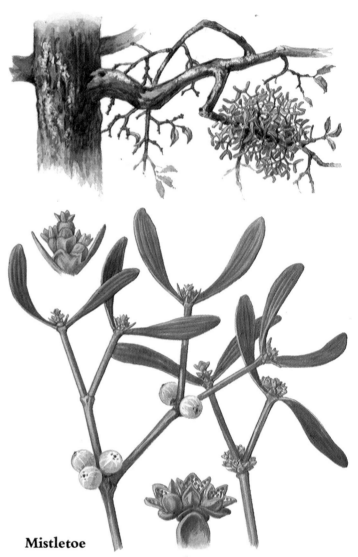

Mistletoe

asking while standing under the hung blossoms at a celebration. In fact, any girl standing under mistletoe is apt to be kissed.

Great Mullein

SCIENTIFIC NAMES: *Verbascum thapsiforme (Verbascum densiflorum)*.

OTHER POPULAR NAME: Aaron's rod.

FAMILY: Scrophulariaceae—Figwort Family.

RANGE: The great mullein stands on stony, pebbly and clayey ground and sunny slopes, street inclines, quarries and refuse dumps all over Europe. Species *thapsiforme* is European; species *thapsus* (common mullein) is native to Europe and Asia but extensively naturalized in North America in old, dry fields and along railways and highways.

DESCRIPTION: This plant, which grows to 2 metres (about 80 inches) tall, got its German name meaning "king's candle" from its candle-straight, tapering, scepter-like growth. On the stalk are leaves that are like white felt on both sides, which become smaller and smaller toward the top of the stalk, with the lower part forming a pyramid, while the upper part is crowned with a candle-like spike of gleaming yellow blossoms. The 5 yellow stamens are divided into two kinds. The 3 upper ones have hairy, somewhat shorter and obliquely set anthers; the 2 lower ones are hairless and of increased length.

ELEMENTS CONTAINED: Up to 11 per cent sugar, fat, a bitter principle, saponin, traces of essential oil, a great deal of mucilage, gum, dye substance, malic and phosphoric acid salts.

MEDICINAL USE: The flowers—*Flores Verbasci*.

A decoction of 5 grams (77 grains avdp) in a cup of water is used externally as an emollient and pain-assuaging application for treatment of ulcers, wounds and external hemorrhoids.

On account of its considerable mucilage content and the simultaneous presence of a bitter principle and saponin, its internal use is indicated in cases of colic conditions and/or relaxation of the digestive tract, as well as in cases of inflamed and mucus-clogged air passages. It also has a beneficial influence on liver and gall troubles.

CULINARY USE: The flowers, which are not hairy like the rest of the plant, can be added to salads.

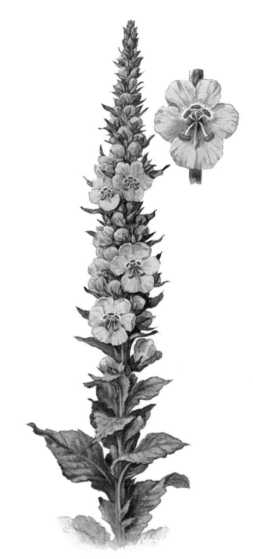

Great Mullein

Mustard

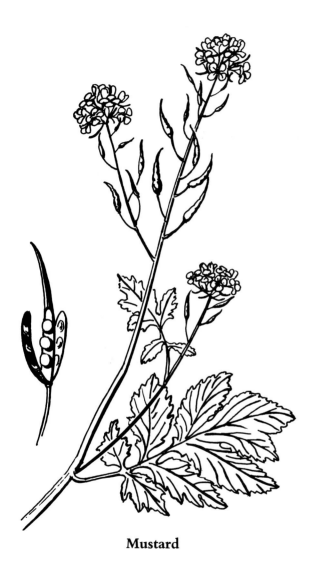

Mustard

SCIENTIFIC NAMES: *Brassica nigra (Sinapis nigra), Brassica alba (Sinapis alba).*

OTHER POPULAR NAMES: Black mustard *(S. nigra),* white mustard *(S. alba).*

FAMILY: Cruciferae—Mustard Family.

RANGE: These two species are natives of Europe and Asia and both are naturalized in North America. They are usually found in fields and open spaces, and along roads and walls.

DESCRIPTION: These two herbs closely resemble one another. Black mustard is an annual, growing to a height of from 3–6 feet (about 1–2 metres), with numerous spreading branches. Its lower leaves are broad and deeply cut, while its upper ones are slender and entire (uncut). The stem and branches are sometimes smooth, but more often covered with rough hairs. The yellow flowers, borne in terminal clusters, have 4 petals, suggesting a cross (hence the name of this plant family—Cruciferae means cross-bearers). The small, dark brown seeds mature in summer. White mustard is similar in appearance, but is a smaller plant, with larger flowers, and larger, light brown seeds.

ELEMENTS CONTAINED: Myrosin (an enzyme), sinigrin (a glucoside), potassium salt, glucose and essential oil (isothiocyanate of allyl). White mustard has a glucoside called sinalbin in place of sinigrin.

MEDICINAL USES: The oil—*Oleum Sinapis volatile.*

It is used in mustard plasters externally. Internally it increases the peristaltic action of the stomach and stimulates salivation, and is used as an emetic.

CULINARY USES: Black mustard seed, ground and mixed with vinegar and spices is widely used as a condiment with meats and in sandwiches, in mayonnaise and other sauces, and in pickles. White mustard leaves are used in salads in Europe, as are the leaves of the very similar *B. juncea* in the Orient and the southern United States (where "mustard greens" are a standard item of diet). The young leaves of the black mustard are also used as a salad in Europe and Asia.

NETTLE

SCIENTIFIC NAME: *Urtica urens* and *dioica*.

OTHER POPULAR NAMES: Stinging nettle. Sp. *dioica*: Great stinging nettle, great nettle, common nettle; Sp. *urens*: small nettle.

FAMILY: Urticaceae—Nettle Family.

RANGE: Worldwide.

DESCRIPTION: These two nettles are found widely in Europe and America. The small smartly stinging nettle *(Urtica urens)* has deep green leaves with saw-toothed edges. This species bears male flowers (stamens) and female (pistils) on the same plant. The large and dioecious (having male and female plants) nettle *(Urtica dioica)* has leaves that are more grey-green. The male plant has long, hanging inflorescences of male flowers, while the female bears only pistillate flowers. *Dioica* does not sting as smartly as *urens* and also a subspecies hardly stings at all.

ELEMENTS CONTAINED: Considerable tannic acid, lecithin, a skin-irritating glycoside, abundant chlorophyll, a comparatively large amount of iron, silicic acid; rich in lime, potassium, phosphorus, sulphur, chlorine, sodium and vitamins A, B and C.

MEDICINAL USE: Leaves—*Folia Urticae*; whole plant—*Herba Urticae*; root—*Radix Urticae*; seeds—*Semen Urticae*.

Owing to its great abundance of iron and chlorophyll, the stinging nettle has an especially good blood-building effect. It also works as a hemostatic agent to stop bleeding and as a blood purifier; it dissolves mucus and acts as an expectorant as well as a diuretic. Taken internally, it helps cure mucous congestion of the chest and lungs, hematemesis (vomiting blood), hemoptysis (spitting up blood from the respiratory tract), hematuria (presence of blood or blood cells in the urine), skin irritations and inflammation of the urinary tract. Internal dosage is given as a tea, 2–4 grams (30.8–61.6 grains avdp). Use both leaves and plant and scald by pouring 1 cup of boiling water over them. The root can also be used to make a light decoction.

Nettle juice is applied externally to promote the growth of hair.

CULINARY USE: Fresh, young nettles are chopped fine and mixed in with curds or salad greens. The young nettles do not sting. They are also effective as a spring tonic.

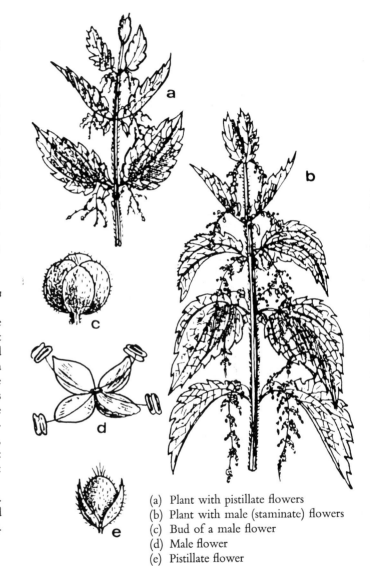

(a) Plant with pistillate flowers
(b) Plant with male (staminate) flowers
(c) Bud of a male flower
(d) Male flower
(e) Pistillate flower

Nettle

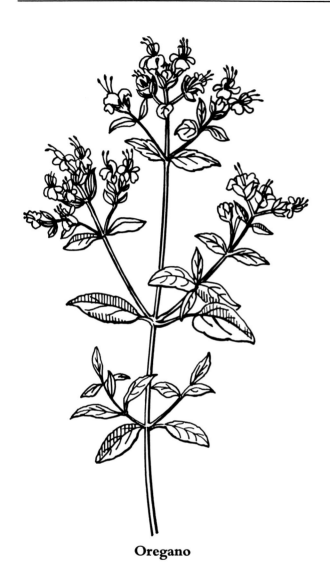

Oregano

OREGANO

SCIENTIFIC NAMES: *Origanum vulgare (Origanum mexicana)*.
OTHER POPULAR NAMES: Mexican sage, Mexican oregano.
FAMILY: Labiatae—Mint Family.
RANGE: Oregano *(Origanum vulgare)* is native to the mountainous terrain around the Mediterranean Sea. The Greeks and Romans carried it into Europe from Palestine and Syria. Brought by the Spaniards to the New World, it is now grown extensively in Mexico as *Origanum mexicana* and is a prized seasoning of the Spanish, Mexicans and Italians, as well as of gourmet cooks throughout the United States, where whole oregano is available on the spice shelves of food stores. Oregano is a perennial herb in warm climates, annual in the north.
DESCRIPTION: From the nearly horizontal root-stock, a stem grows upward about 77 cm (2½ feet), bearing the pungent leaves and flowering tops that are used for seasoning. The leaves are broadly oval in shape, 4 cm (1½ inches) long. The flowers grow in 5 cm wide (2 inch) clusters.
ELEMENT CONTAINED: An essential oil called origanum oil.
MEDICINAL USE: The leaves—*Folia Origani*.

In folk medicine, it was recommended that the leaves be chewed for toothache. The dried leaves mixed with honey were applied as a salve to bruises and contusions. Oregano tea is taken as a stomachic and for loss of appetite.
CULINARY USE: Similar to marjoram, but more intense and stronger in taste and aroma.

Use chopped, fresh leaves or dried, whole oregano. Sprinkle on all kinds of meats, liver and similar dishes; add to shrimp salad, potato salad, green salads, fowl stuffing. Cooked with peas, beans, greens, tomatoes, soups, scrambled eggs, omelets and added to boiled egg dishes, oregano gives a piquancy of taste. Especially useful for spicing Italian, Spanish and Mexican dishes, particularly spaghetti sauces, chili, hamburgers, toasted cheese sandwiches, creamed and hash-brown potatoes, and on pizza.

Pansy

SCIENTIFIC NAME: *Viola tricolor.*

OTHER POPULAR NAMES: Wild pansy, heart's-ease, field pansy, garden pansy, Johnny Jump-up, stepmother.

RANGE: Everywhere in Europe we find this flower on meadows, fallow land, along the shady edges of woods, on the arid soil of roadsides. It is naturalized in parts of eastern North America.

DESCRIPTION: This undemanding, storm- and sun-defying little plant occurs in many forms. Sometimes it is hairy, sometimes smooth; here the leaves are stemmed and roundish, there long, heart-shaped, or even blunt; often slightly notched. And on the very next plant are lyre-shaped, pinnate leaves and heart-shaped wide ones. The stem is partly procumbent, partly erect, and the flowers vary among yellow, blue, violet and white, and most bear all these shades in various arrangements.

ELEMENTS CONTAINED: Rich in saponin; mucilage, tannin, methyl salycilate (artificial oil of wintergreen), flavone, glycoside, viola quercitrine; in the ashes, mainly lime and magnesium salts.

MEDICINAL USE: The blooming plant—*Herba Violae tricoloris.*

A decoction of the pansy plant helps externally. (Boil 1 tablespoonful of the plant for a short time in 1 cup of water, allow it to stand 10 minutes, then strain.) It is used against milk-crust (vesicular eczema occurring on the face and scalp of nursing infants) in children, eczema-like and scrofula-like skin eruptions.

Internally, the tea (1 tablespoonful of the plant scalded with 1 cup of boiling water, or allowed to soak in cold water overnight) has a diaphoretic and diuretic effect, loosens phlegm, and is a mild laxative. For this reason it is a good blood-purifying agent and is effective against a surplus of uric acid, rheumatism, gout, catarrh of the stomach and intestines, mucous diarrhea, and catarrh of the bladder. Colds are also within its sphere of use.

CULINARY USE: None.

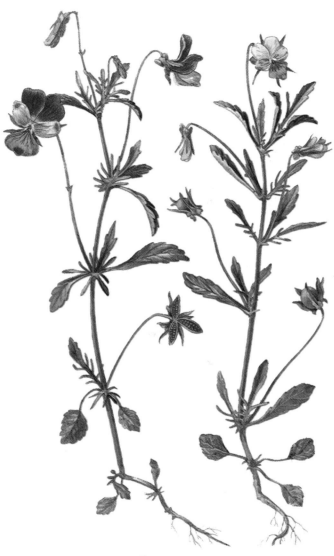

Pansy

Parsley

SCIENTIFIC NAMES: *Petroselinum hortense (P. crispum, P. sativum, Carum petroselinum).*

OTHER POPULAR NAMES: Rock parsley, common parsley, carum.

FAMILY: Umbelliferae—Parsley or Carrot Family.

RANGE: This plant, which is native to the lands southeast of the Mediterranean Sea and in northwestern Africa, has spread everywhere today and is grown in gardens as a seasoning plant.

DESCRIPTION: Like many Umbelliferae, this biennial plant forms in its first year only the carrot-like, whitish root and a leaf rosette. Not until the second year does the sharp-edged, erect stalk spring up, with pinnate leaves along it, becoming simpler toward the top. The umbels bear small, greenish-yellow blossoms.

ELEMENTS CONTAINED: All parts of the plant but especially the fruits, have an essential oil, which contains the poisonous apiole. In addition, mineral substances are contained in diverse quantities in the plant parts (especially manganese and in the seeds, some iron), and the glycoside, apiin.

MEDICINAL USE: The plant—*Herba Petroselini*; seeds—*Semen Petroselini*; fruits—*Fructus Petroselini*; root—*Radix Petroselini*.

The fruits of the parsley are said to be deadly to birds, and in human beings as well they can damage the liver cell tissue. For this reason, one should take the fruit and seeds only on the advice of a physician. The essential oil is used most frequently as an abortifacient and is acknowledged as an aphrodisiac. It is a powerful diuretic agent, has a beneficial effect on bladder and kidney stones and rheumatism, and is also used in cases of stoppage of the urine accompanying prostate trouble. The root is popular for use as a spice (see below). As a digestive stimulant, it counteracts gastritis, as well as over-activity of the thyroid gland.

CULINARY USE: Root and leaves are usable, not the fruit or seeds. The root may be boiled with other foods, but never boil the fresh leaves. Smooth leaves are spicier than curled; dry and use them fine-chopped.

Use in soups, sauces, with meat, vegetables, in stews, noodle and rice dishes, salad, herb-butter, curds and cheese dishes, with eggs, omelets and soufflés, potato dishes.

Fresh, green parsley is rich in vitamin C and builds blood. It can also be deep-frozen and kept as an always green supply.

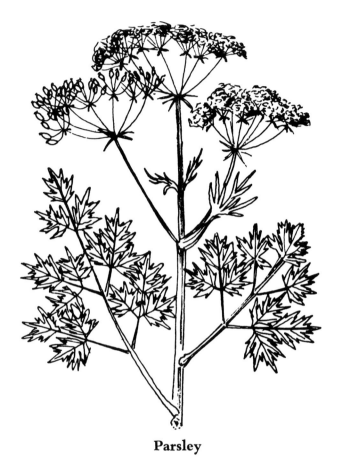

Parsley

Peppermint

SCIENTIFIC NAME: *Mentha piperita.*

OTHER POPULAR NAMES: Lammint, brandy mint.

FAMILY: Labiatae—Mint Family.

RANGE: Peppermint grows everywhere in the temperate zones, and is cultivated in many countries. It likes light and moisture.

DESCRIPTION: The knee-high plant bears numerous opposed, oval, sharp-pointed, saw-toothed leaves, from the axes of which grow pseudo-spikes of small, violet blossoms.

ELEMENTS CONTAINED: The constituent most present is essential oil, in quantity up to 2 per cent, and anywhere from 5 per cent to 90 per cent menthol and 8 per cent to 20 per cent menthone. In addition, tannin, a bitter principle, oxydase and catalase are present.

MEDICINAL USE: The leaves—*Folia Menthae piperitae.*

Probably, in every household, next to chamomile, you are likely to find peppermint, yet how few people know how to use this important medicinal plant. It is often drunk as a household tea, but in doing so, it should not be forgotten that peppermint is a medicinal plant which can be harmful in regular use, even if taken in the prescribed preparation mixtures. Peppermint tea should be drunk in daily use only in extreme dilution and varied with other herb teas.

Peppermint is used externally in the form of ordinary peppermint oil, as a rub for topical pains, neuralgia and headache.

Internally, the plant has a stimulating effect on the metabolism, being at the same time antispasmodic and an agent for worming through the digestive tract. It loosens uterine cramps, itensifies menses and potency, and is recommended for strengthening the nerves. In cases of gall-bladder colic, the tea resolves the cramping condition.

CULINARY USE: Peppermint tea is very popular (see above). It is also used in candy-making. The leaves are sometimes used as a seasoning, and the essence is used to make peppermint liqueur.

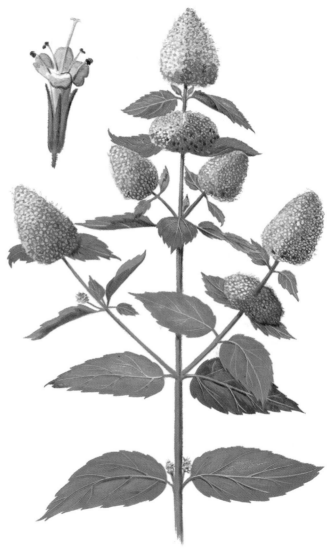

Peppermint

Plantain

SCIENTIFIC NAME: *Plantago major.*

OTHER POPULAR NAME: Greater plantain.

FAMILY: Plantaginaceae—Plantain Family.

RANGE: Plantain is found throughout the world, along streets and roadsides, on meadows and fields, as well as in lawns.

DESCRIPTION: Everybody is familiar with this rosette of leaves that even grows between paving stones and on well-travelled ways, and is very hard to uproot. Each wide leaf of the rosette is shot through with 7 veins, while from the middle of the plant grows a flower spike that does not reveal its full beauty except upon close inspection. The plantain follows mankind into all regions of the earth. Its small seeds are enclosed in a gelatinous pod which, in wet weather, sticks to the feet of people and animals, and so gets distributed widely. For this reason, the Indians called the plantain, "white man's foot."

ELEMENTS CONTAINED: Tannic acid, a bitter principle, and mucilage.

MEDICINAL USE: The leaves—*Folia Plantaginis majoris.*

It is an ancient custom to lay crushed plantain leaves on new wounds. They have a cooling and pain-relieving effect where skin has been galled or abraded.

Plantain is given internally as a tea; 2–4 grams (1–2 level tablespoonfuls) of the dried leaves, scalded with 1 cup of boiling water, or boil briefly. It is a help in cases of mucous catarrh of the lungs, intermittent fever, hemorrhoids, hemorrhages, blennorrhea (discharge of mucus), and abscesses or ulcers.

CULINARY USE: Plantain is said to have formerly been eaten as a pot-herb in the Orient.

(a) Flower (enlarged)

Plantain

LANCE-LEAF PLANTAIN

SCIENTIFIC NAME: *Plantago lanceolata*.

OTHER POPULAR NAMES: Ribwort plantain, cocks-and-hens, rib-grass, soldiers' herb.

FAMILY: Plantaginaceae—Plantain Family.

RANGE: Like the greater plantain *(Plantago major)*, this species grows everywhere along roads, fences, the edges of woods, and in meadows and is a nuisance in lawns. It can also be seen in city sidewalks, growing in cracks in the pavement.

DESCRIPTION: Out of the short root-stock grows a rosette of leaves close to the ground and which is distinguished from that of the greater plantain by longer and narrower leaves with never more than 3 to 5 veins. Also, the leafless flower stem is not smooth but furrowed, and the inconspicuous flowers bear 4 filaments that hang far outside, whose pollen sacs are yellow and not violet as in the greater plantain. Between these two species, there is an intermediate species *(Plantago media)* with elliptical leaves and pinkish-red pollen sacs. Of the many other species one with narrow, grass-like leaves is found in mountainous areas.

ELEMENTS CONTAINED: A bitter glycoside (aucubin), mucilage, silicic acid, xanthophyll, enzymes, vitamin C, tannin, mineral salts.

MEDICINAL USE: The leaves—*Folia Plantaginis*.

Lance-leaf plantain is one of the best known medicinal plants. As with greater plantain, the crushed leaves are laid on fresh, bleeding, abraded wounds. Badly healing old wounds, scabs, and eczema are similarly treated.

For internal use, lance-leaf plantain is valued as a cough remedy. In cases of catarrh of the upper air passages, whooping cough, catarrh of the apex of the lungs, even in asthma and light cases of tuberculosis, this medicinal plant is helpful. Because of its silicic acid content, lance-leaf plantain has a diuretic effect and for this reason is used for bladder trouble and stone complaints of the kidneys and bladder. Its effectiveness as an antispasmodic, stomachic, and blood purifier is also well known.

CULINARY USE: None.

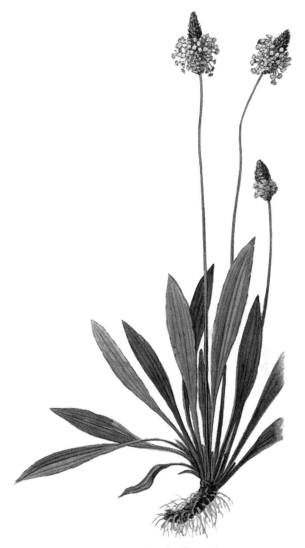

Lance-leaf Plantain

COMMON POLYPODY

SCIENTIFIC NAME: *Polypodium vulgare.*

OTHER POPULAR NAMES: Beech polypody, wall-fern, female fern, fern root, rock brake, rock polypody, brake root.

FAMILY: Polypodiaceae—Common-Fern Family.

RANGE: Common polypody thrives in Europe in rock crevices, by old walls, in ruins and shady forests. In western North America, a variety, *P. occidentale*, ranges from California to Alaska; variety *hesperium* from British Columbia to California.

DESCRIPTION: From a thick, woody, creeping root-stock, sprout bright green leaves, which are rolled up at first, then unfold gradually into imposing fronds. These simple, feathery leaves, which even last through the winter, have golden yellow sporangia on their undersides, arranged in two rows.

ELEMENTS CONTAINED: Tannic acid, an abundance of mucilage, sugar, resin, fat oil, glycyrrhizin (glycyrrhizic acid).

MEDICINAL USE: The root-stock—*Rhizoma Polypodii.*

The tea is made by pouring scalding water over 4–10 grams (62–154 grains avdp) of the finely chopped root-stock. Do not boil, since boiling destroys the glycyrrhizin. The tea is used in cases of disease of the air passages, especially catarrhal cough and bronchitis. However, common polypody also has a beneficial effect on other diseases, such as gout, swelling of the glands and chronic constipation, as well as disorders of the spleen and liver.

CULINARY USE: The young shoots of polypody may be prepared and eaten in the same manner as those of the male fern (see p. 94).

Common Polypody

CORN POPPY

SCIENTIFIC NAME: *Papaver rhoeas.*

OTHER POPULAR NAMES: Field poppy, Shirley poppy, common red poppy.

FAMILY: Papaveraceae—Poppy Family.

RANGE: The corn poppy is known throughout Europe as a field weed, and has been naturalized in North America. It grows on uncultivated ground such as slopes and declivities, field borders, and vineyards.

DESCRIPTION: The flowers of the 4 wild species of poppy gleam a bright red among the lush green of young standing crops. The *Papaver rhoeas* grows the largest flower. On a slender stem it grows upward, leaving incised, longish leaves behind it. The entire plant is slender. The buds hang down. Not until the blossoms unfold do they stand half erect. The flower is everything with this plant, but its deep red bloom does not last long. A breath of wind and the 4 petals with blue-black bases fall off. Their fire fades on the ground, while the dry capsule towers stiffly into the air. The milky sap of the native poppy has none of the poisonous character of the cultivated *Papaver somniferum.*

ELEMENTS CONTAINED: Gum, fat, tannin, starch, wax, resin, a harmless alkaloid, rheadine (rhoeadine), rheadine acid, corn poppy acid, red dye substance.

MEDICINAL USE: Flowers—*Flores Rhoeados.*

Corn poppy tea used to be given to small children as a sedative, a practice that is still continued today in many regions. Modern science has also discovered that, next to its sedative effect, corn poppy also gives a stimulating impulse to the metabolism.

CULINARY USE: In France, the leaves are sometimes cooked and served like spinach, even though they have a slight narcotic effect.

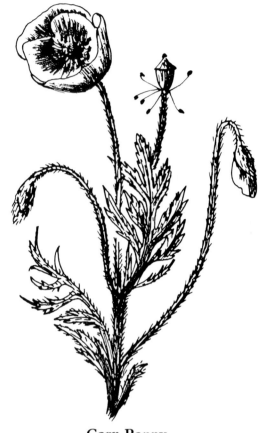

Corn Poppy

POT MARIGOLD

SCIENTIFIC NAME: *Calendula officinalis.*

OTHER POPULAR NAMES: Common pot marigold, marygold, old marigold, marigold, calendula, marybud, holigold.

FAMILY: Compositae—Composite Family.

RANGE: This sun-loving, medicinal plant is native to the Mediterranean region. In the Middle Ages, in temperate latitudes, it was cultivated everywhere in farm gardens. Nowadays it occurs outdoors in gardens as well as occasionally growing wild and is cultivated in many districts as a medicinal plant. It is a popular flower-garden plant and grown for cut flowers in winter.

The garden marigolds called French and African belong to the genus Tagetes, and in the United States, have usurped the name marigold from the calendula, which is less common there.

DESCRIPTION: From the seed, which has a peanut-like shell, sprouts a heavily branching stalk with fleshy, softly-haired leaves that mount up toward the branched inflorescence with its golden-yellow to orange composite flowers, of which the ray flowers alone bear fruit, while the disc flowers are barren. Quickly fading away, they make a place for new, yellow blooms. If one picks a flower, a remarkable smell of putrefaction remains on the hand, derived from a resin.

ELEMENTS CONTAINED: Essential oil, a carotin-related dyestuff, a bitter principle, nitrogen-containing mucilage, resin, gum, calendulin.

MEDICINAL USE: The blossoms—*Flores Calendulae*; the plant—*Herba Calendulae*.

An alcohol extract of the calendula, diluted with water, is used in cases of crushed, old, inflamed, suppurating and lacerated, gaping wounds, where arnica would only be harmful. Formerly, such an extract was even used for carcinomas of the breasts and the uterus. According to Kneipp, a salve made from it is used today for lacerated wounds, ulcers, burns and sunburn.

Internally, calendula as a tea made from 2–4 grams (30.8–61.6 grains avdp) scalded with 1 cup of boiling water is beneficially effective in treatment of stomach ulcers, phlebitis, inflamed and swollen glandular organs, such as in swelling of the liver or the spleen.

In cosmetic manufacture, calendula is known as an additive to face creams.

CULINARY USE: The petals of this plant have been used in cookery as a substitute for saffron, as a seasoning for soups and stews, and to give a yellow tint to butter.

The petals of the *Tagetes* genus are sometimes used in the same way.

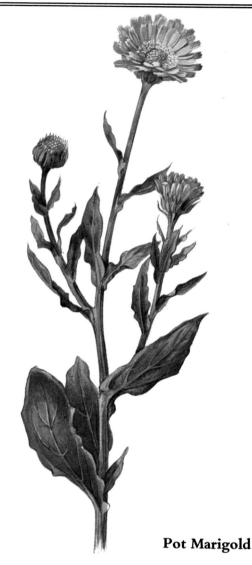

Pot Marigold

RESTHARROW

SCIENTIFIC NAME: *Ononis spinosa.*

OTHER POPULAR NAMES: Spinous restharrow, petty whin, cammock, stay plough.

FAMILY: Leguminosae—Pea or Pulse Family.

RANGE: Restharrow, native to Europe, grows on barren fields, along roads and on sterile slopes.

DESCRIPTION: The deeply penetrating root, according to botanists, keeps reaching downward until it comes upon lime-bearing soil. By collecting and storing lime and nitrogen, the plant improves the poor soils in which it alone grows. Fertilizing drives it out at once and makes it unnecessary to pull the plants out of the ground. Generally, this task is so difficult that long ago, weeding farm women created their own expressions of curse and anger to utter. The above-ground part of the plant appears as a mean, thorn-beset shrub adorned with large, pink blossoms which shimmer with a violet hue, thanks to their blue veins.

ELEMENTS CONTAINED: Some essential oil, fat oil, sugar, gum, starch, resin, tannin, citric acid, glycosides and ononine.

MEDICINAL USE: The root—*Radix Ononidis.*

The main effect of restharrow is diuretic. The tea made from 2–4 grams (30.8–61.6 grains avdp) of the root are scalded by pouring 1 cup of boiling water over them; or, they may be briefly boiled, however, the tea loses its effect soon and therefore a respite should be taken after about 3 days. The uric acid surplus of the body is reduced by this medicinal plant, and for this reason, restharrow is included in tea-mixtures taken for gout and rheumatism. Flushing of the kidneys has a beneficial effect on gravel, catarrh of the bladder, weakness of the bladder, and dropsy.

CULINARY USE: None.

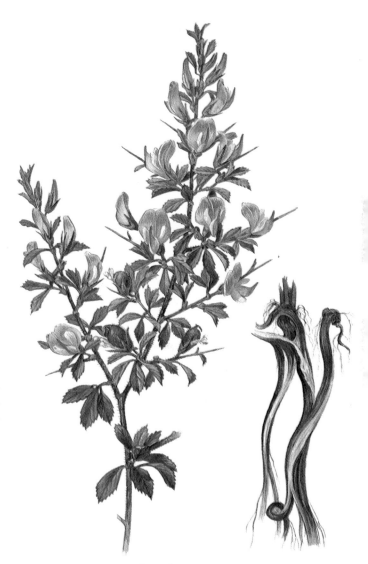

Restharrow

ROSEMARY

SCIENTIFIC NAME: *Rosmarinus officinalis*.

OTHER POPULAR NAMES: Wild rosemary, marsh rosemary, moorwort.

FAMILY: Labiatae—Mint Family.

RANGE: Rosemary is native to the coasts around the Mediterranean Sea. In Europe (and America as well) it thrives in gardens.

DESCRIPTION: This spread-out, bushy subshrub with evergreen, needle-like leaves grows man-high (up to 2 metres or 6 feet). For a short time in the spring, the plant produces small bright violet blossoms on the young shoots.

ELEMENTS CONTAINED: Essential oil which contains camphor-like substances, tannin, a bitter principle, and resin.

MEDICINAL USE: The leaves—*Folia Rosmarini*; oil—*Oleum Rosmarini*.

In the Middle Ages, this plant was brought over the Alps into northern Europe and was soon very well liked as a pot and a garden herb. All kinds of folk customs became attached to the spicy redolent plant, from which were broken sprigs for baptisms, marriages and funerals. Kneipp became acquainted with the plant in this wise in Swabia (Germany), and he included it among his most used medicinal plants, probably on account of its wide range of use.

Rosemary is a stimulant for the circulation and the nerves. It does not work directly on the heart, but through the central nervous system. Externally, it has a tonic effect in 10-minute baths at normal body temperature—37° C. (98.6° F.)—followed by a half-hour of bed rest in circulatory and nervous troubles, conditions of exhaustion after excessive intellectual demands, and low blood pressure. These soothing baths should, however, be taken only in the morning or the forenoon, because their stimulating effect could do little to promote sleep.

Rosemary is dispensed by drops for internal use. These affect the tension of the blood vessels and nerves to allow blood pressure that is too high to lower and, if too low, to rise. The drops also help conquer fatigue and beneficially influence productive power, animate the circulation, stimulate the metabolism, restore good blood circulation, and combat diabetes. Elderly people should take rosemary to stimulate their systems.

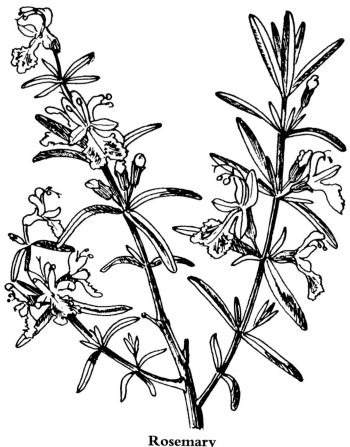

Rosemary

CULINARY USE: Harshly spicy, camphor-like aroma and taste. Fresh: Chop young tip-shoots fine. Dried: Use cut or ground.

Use with meat and game dishes (especially lamb), in the preparation of sausage, soups, sauces, stews, fish, mushroom and potato dishes, as well as with tomato soup, egg dishes, salads. It has a strengthening effect on the stomach and circulatory system, calms the nerves and combats rheumatism.

For tea: Take 1 teaspoonful, and pour over it 1 cup of boiling water.

Sage

SCIENTIFIC NAME: *Salvia officinalis*.

OTHER POPULAR NAMES: Red sage, white sage, garden sage, wild sage.

FAMILY: Labiatae—Mint Family.

RANGE: Sage abounds on the bare limestone cliffs of Dalmatia; on the slopes of Greece, the Balkans and Spain. Everywhere else, however, it is found in cultivation. (The sage found in the western parts of the United States is not the same plant, but a species of Artemisia.)

DESCRIPTION: Harsh and bitter, the aroma of sage climbs upward like a cloud of smoke. Up to a metre (40 inches) high, the sub-shrub has a square stem, woody below with thick, wrinkled leaves which are almost spear-shaped and which stand directly opposed to each other. Blue inflorescences rise up from the profusion of leaves, bearing large flowers which are an ideal fit for the bee's body.

ELEMENTS CONTAINED: 2 per cent essential oil, 5 per cent tannin, 6 per cent starch, 5.6 per cent resin, phosphoric-acid salts and traces of nitric acid, and salts of potash and lime.

MEDICINAL USE: The leaves—*Folia Salviae*.

Sage is used as a gargle for inflammation of the mouth and throat.

People of the Middle Ages took it internally as an invigorating agent. Today, sage leaves are used to counteract night sweats of pulmonary disease victims. *Salvia officinalis* also has a beneficial effect upon the digestive tract, inflammatory processes of the air passages, the female organs where the pelvis is small, and liver troubles.

As a tea, it is effective against troubles of the gums: Pour 1 cup boiling water over 1 teaspoonful, and use cold.

CULINARY USE: Strongly aromatic with a slight taste of nutmeg. When used fresh, chop it fine. When dried, use it whole or pulverized. It can spice vegetables, one-dish meals, legumes, liver, kidney, fowl, game, fish. When dried, it has a very strong aroma.

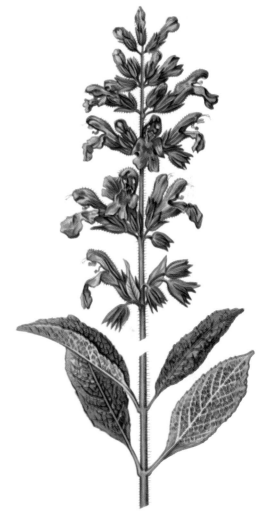

Sage

St. John's-Wort

SCIENTIFIC NAME: *Hypericum perforatum.*

OTHER POPULAR NAMES: Perforated St. John's-wort, common hypericum, All-Saints-wort, John's wort.

FAMILY: Hypericaceae—St. John's-wort Family.

RANGE: St. John's-wort blooms everywhere in Europe on sunny slopes and inclines and at the edges of woods, and grows abundantly in America, where it has been naturalized. It proves very annoying to farmers everywhere.

DESCRIPTION: The plant got the name St. John's-wort because it contains a red resin in small, black glands within its golden-yellow blossoms. If you rub the petals between your fingers, this red resin comes out and makes your fingers red. In the Middle Ages, there was a saying that the plant sprang from the blood shed by St. John the Baptist when he was beheaded. Therefore, it is often blessed by a priest and worn to ward off disease and temptations. The devil is supposed to have perforated the leaves of St. John's-wort with thousands of tiny needle punctures, hoping to make them wither. These tiny, translucent holes can still be seen by holding the smooth, oval leaflets up to the light. They are filled with a pure essential oil.

The plant grows about knee-high. The leaflets stand opposed on angular stems, and from the angle at the bases of the leaflets at the tip of the stem spring the golden corymbs (erect clusters).

ELEMENTS CONTAINED: Red and yellow dyes, easily soluble in alcohol, are found in the flowers. Moreover, the plant contains essential oil, a glycoside, tannin, flavone, pectin, choline, pentosane, stearine, palmitine (a glyceride of palmitic acid), myristic acid, phlobaphene, and mineral substances.

MEDICINAL USE: The plant with flowers—*Herba Hyperici.*

Used externally, St. John's-wort oil is an exceptional remedy for the healing of wounds. It is recommended by modern medicine as a slow but enduring tranquilizer which has no side effects as do synthetic agents. A tea is made of 2–4 grams (30.8–61.6 grains advp) scalded by pouring 1 cup of boiling water over the herb. When this is drunk for a period of 10 days, or the well known red oil (oleic acid) is taken, a distinct lightening of mood is effected. In order to obtain a lasting effect, the treatment should be continued for several weeks longer.

St. John's-wort has a photo-sensitizing effect. One should not expose oneself to the sun during the course of treatment, as

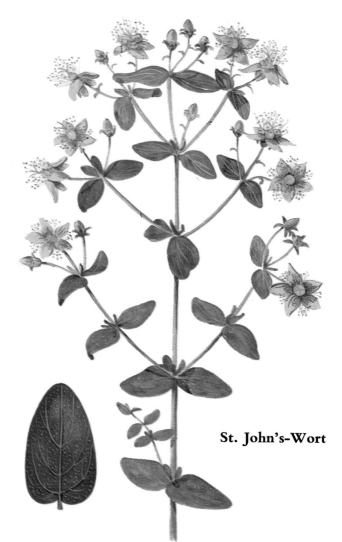

St. John's-Wort

sunburn will quickly result, against which St. John's-wort oil again is used with success. The tranquilizing effect certainly derives from the fact that St. John's-wort aids the functioning of the liver and strengthens the nerves.

CULINARY USE: None.

SANICLE

SCIENTIFIC NAMES: *Sanicula europaea; Sanicula marilandica* (American).

OTHER POPULAR NAMES: Wood sanicle, black snakeroot, pool root.

FAMILY: Umbelliferae—Parsley or Carrot Family.

RANGE: The European wood sanicle prefers growing in the half-shade of deciduous forests, in soil that is rich in humus and lime. It is spread throughout Europe, Asia and North Africa.

The American sanicle is indigenous to and common in the United States and Canada, where it is found in low woods and thickets, flowering in June.

DESCRIPTION: The perennial root-stock lies almost horizontal in the ground. It has many runners and grows ground-leaves with 5 lobes and long stems. Every year, a flower-bearing sprout shoots up, which has only a few leaves and these grow smaller and simpler as they mount toward the top. The little umbels form radiating balls with white or reddish blossoms on long umbel-stems, which bloom in May and June. Also, the fruits show the radiating form with their bent, soft thorns.

ELEMENTS CONTAINED: A plentiful amount of lime and silicic acid; in addition, saponin, tannin, essential oil, resin and a bitter principle.

MEDICINAL USE: The plant—*Herba Saniculae*; root—*Radix Saniculae*.

A tea of the sanicle plant made from 1 gram (15.4 grains avdp) scalded with 1 cup of boiling water, or sanicle root made from 1 gram (15.4 grains avdp) put into 1 cup of water and boiled for a short time is used for compresses on bruises, sprains, suppurating wounds, and ulcers. Sanicle has long been known and highly prized for its wound-healing properties, since this plant is hemostatic (blood-stanching), cleans out suppurating wounds, and stimulates healing.

Used internally, the tea stops bleeding from the stomach, intestine, lungs and bladder. Also, inflammation of the digestive tract is beneficially influenced.

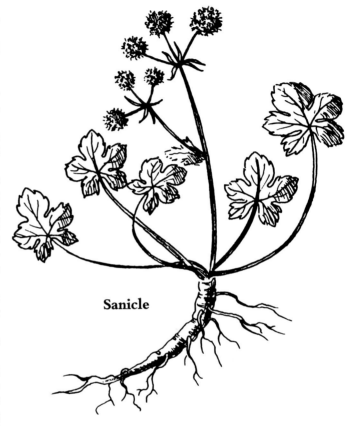

Sanicle

S. marilandica: Domestically, it is used with advantage in throat irritation and is beneficially employed in various other conditions. Add a teaspoonful of the root, cut small or granulated, to a cup of boiling water. Drink cold, one cupful per day, in large gulps.

CULINARY USE: None.

Summer Savory

SUMMER SAVORY

SCIENTIFIC NAME: *Satureja hortensis* (formerly *Satureia*).

OTHER POPULAR NAMES: Bean herb, Bohnenkraut.

FAMILY: Labiatae—Mint Family.

RANGE: This plant, widely known as a kitchen herb, is native to the eastern part of the Mediterranean region, and is also found in the eastern part of the United States. We do not find it mentioned anywhere by the Greeks, but it was highly esteemed by the ancient Romans. Today it is grown in gardens and fields.

DESCRIPTION: From a heavily branched root, the annual plant develops a bushy, multi-branched stalk that grows to a height of 20–30 cm (about 8–12 inches). The stem is tough and covered with short hairs and attached to it are practically stemless, short-haired, dark-green entire leaves which, like the stem part when it is still young, are possessed of oil-bags. The white, pink and soft violet flowers bloom from July into October and form false spikes in the upper leaf axils.

ELEMENTS CONTAINED: About 2 per cent essential oil and 4 to 8 per cent tannic acid.

MEDICINAL USE: The whole plant when in flower—*Herba Saturejae*. Summer savory is known in folk medicine.and homeopathy as a remedy for diarrhea, colic and disturbances of the digestive tract.

CULINARY USE: It is used as a seasoning for beans and other legumes, as well as for various kinds of cabbage, because it eliminates the gas-forming effect of these vegetables. It also finds use in sausage-making and in meat dishes.

It has a strongly aromatic smell and a pepper-like taste. Harvest before blooming. Use the stem along with the rest of the plant, but remove after cooking. Use fresh in bunches, dried or ground. Summer savory should only be allowed to soak (draw or steep) in the food.

This seasoning is used with potato and mushroom dishes, and mutton and it may be put into various salads, such as cucumber, green bean and head lettuce and is also added to sauerkraut, soufflés and ragouts. When dried, it should be kept in a well-sealed container.

It mitigates the smell of cooking cabbage.

SCABIOUS

SCIENTIFIC NAMES: *Succisa pratensis (Scabiosa succisa, S. arvensis).*

OTHER POPULAR NAMES: Devil's bit, primrose scabious, horse-weed, daisy fleabane (United States).

FAMILY: Dipsaceae—Teasel Family.

RANGE: In damp meadows and forest clearings, the scabious is widespread throughout central Europe, especially in Germany.

DESCRIPTION: The short, brown and firm root-stock about 1 cm ($\frac{3}{8}$ inch) thick, is covered with adventitious roots. The plant sends toward the light a rosette of elliptical, mostly whole-edged leaves, from which spring simple or branched flower stems which usually bear smaller and pointed leaves on the branches. The flower heads consist of compact, round masses of small, blue-violet, also blue and occasionally white, flowers.

ELEMENTS CONTAINED: The most important constituents are tannin and a bitter extractive substance; moreover, a small quantity of starch, saponin, and a glycoside.

MEDICINAL USE: The root—*Radix Morsus Diaboli*; plant—*Herba Succisae.*

So-named, scabious is supposed to be a remedy for scabies, an itch caused by mites.

A decoction made from 1–3 grams (15.4–46.2 grains avdp) taken from the root and boiled briefly in 1 cup of water, is used externally for cleaning and healing wounds, similar to arnica.

A tea made of the finely-chopped root from 1–3 grams (15.4–46.2 grains avdp) scalded with 1 cup of boiling water, if taken internally, is beneficial in cases of diarrhea, intestinal and maggot worms. A tea made from the plant is also helpful against liver and gall-bladder troubles.

CULINARY USE: Scabious leaves may be cooked and served like spinach or used raw in salads. Either way they are tasty.

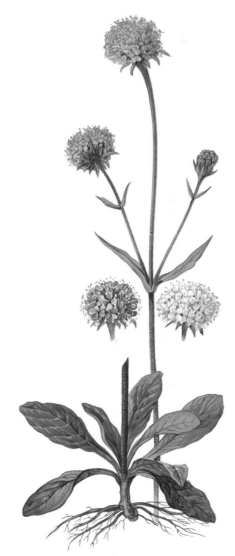

Scabious

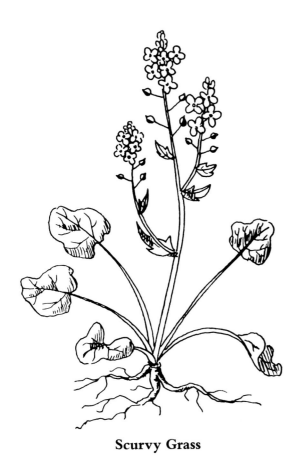

Scurvy Grass

Scurvy Grass

SCIENTIFIC NAME: *Cochlearia officinalis.*

OTHER POPULAR NAMES: Common scurvy grass, spoonwort.

FAMILY: Cruciferae—Mustard Family.

RANGE: This salt-loving plant grows particularly on the beaches of the coasts of western Europe and up into the far north, in arctic North America, and on the Siberian coast. It is also found in the vicinity of salt pits as well as near springs and streams.

DESCRIPTION: This winter-hardy plant, which can be harvested green in the hardest frost, even when the leaves are covered with a crust of ice, springs from the soil with a ground-rosette of long-stemmed, whole-edged, spoon-like leaves on a many-filamented root-stock. In the spring, a sprout shoots upward, the few leaves of which, by weak indentations, bear witness to a disposition toward articulation.

On the ends of the upper, branched shoots stand loose, white flower clusters. In the autumn, this vigorous plant again puts forth flowers, and information comes from Siberia that species growing there which are surprised by frost and snow become frozen in throughout the winter and bloom again in the spring.

ELEMENTS CONTAINED: A large quantity of very stable vitamin C, glycoside, butyl mustard oil, a bitter principle, tannin.

MEDICINAL USE: The plant—*Herba Cochleariae.*

Long before its high content of vitamin C was known, scurvy grass in olden days was being taken along on sea voyages, preserved in brine, for use against scurvy.

Scurvy grass helps quickly to overcome spring fever and fatigue following great physical exertion. It has a hemostatic (blood-stanching) effect on tissues in the mouth and nostrils. The dried plant is a good diuretic in dropsy and salt-dissolving in gout and rheumatism. It has an equally beneficial effect on stoppage of the urine and the formation of calculus.

CULINARY USE: None. (Sometimes grown as a salad vegetable but tastes too much like tar to be liked by many people.)

SESAME

SCIENTIFIC NAMES: *Sesamum indicum* or *Sesamum orientale*.
OTHER POPULAR NAMES: Benne (the word means "grain"), bene, oil-plant, vangloe, tilseed, teel, teel-seed, gingili.
FAMILY: Pedaliaceae—Pedalium Family.
RANGE: Native to the Oriental tropics, sesame is easy to grow in a sunny garden. It is planted in May and harvested in early autumn. The seed pods are cut on the plant before they dry so that they will burst open.
DESCRIPTION: Sesame is an East Indian erect, annual herb well known to the ancients. It was used by the Babylonians and the ancient Sumerians to season wine. In India and Egypt, the oil pressed from sesame seed was used for food, as it was by the Greeks and Romans and still is in the Orient. It is also an ingredient of some margarines.

The plant grows 77–92 cm ($2\frac{1}{2}$–3 feet) high, with oblong or lanceolate leaves, sometimes triple-lobed, up to 13 cm (5 inches) long. The 25-mm-long (inch-long) flowers are pink or white, with short upper lobes.
ELEMENTS CONTAINED: From the seeds is pressed a fat oil called sesame oil, gingelly oil, or teel oil, consisting mainly of sesamol (a crystalline phenolic ether) and sesamolin (a crystalline cyclic ether), which is a powerful agent used in pyrethrum insecticides.
MEDICINAL USE: The leaves—*Folia Sesami*.

For external use, as a tea, the leaves of the sesame plant soothe inflamed or abraded mucous membranes of the mouth and throat. As a poultice or compress, they have an emollient (softening) effect.
CULINARY USE: The seeds are sprinkled on the top of bread, rolls, etc., before baking. They are also used in making certain kinds of sweets, such as halvah, and yield an oil used in making margarine.

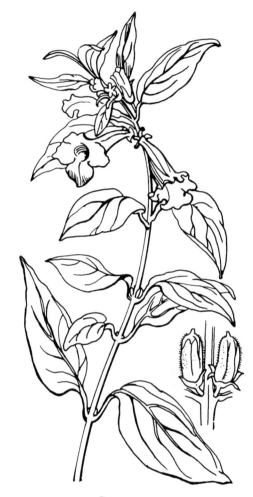

Sesame

Shepherd's Purse

SHEPHERD'S PURSE

SCIENTIFIC NAMES: *Capsella bursa-pastoris (Bursa bursa-pastoris)*.

OTHER POPULAR NAMES: Capsell, shepherd's heart.

FAMILY: Cruciferae—Mustard Family.

RANGE: Shepherd's purse has spread out in all directions from Europe and grows on fields and fallow lands, along roadsides, ditches, slopes, and on heaps of earth.

DESCRIPTION: Practically everyone remembers from childhood the little, heart-shaped pods on a long stalk, growing from a luxuriant rosette of leaves fastened to the earth by a sturdy taproot. The leaves of the rosette are usually more or less divided, but are often undivided. The white blossoms are inconspicuous and in many species, they lack petals entirely, or are transformed into stigmata, so that 10 stigmata are then present instead of 6. Propagation is carried on abundantly and from March into November, shepherd's purses are blooming, fruit-producing and germinating.

ELEMENTS CONTAINED: Potassium, calcium, and sodium salts, allyl isothiocyanate (mustard gas or allyl mustard oil, a poison gas). The presence of choline is conditional on the presence of a fungus.

MEDICINAL USE: The whole plant—*Herba Bursae pastoris*.

Shepherd's purse is dispensed in cases of disease of the kidney ducts and in the occurrence of kidney gravel. Its hemostatic (blood-stanching) effect, its rhythmic impulse upon the sexual region of women, and its influence on the peristaltic action of the bowels are, according to latest research, probably to be traced only to the presence of the fungus. To be sure, it occurs frequently on the plant, but not always.

CULINARY USE: Shepherd's purse was used as a pot-herb in Europe in former times and is still so used in parts of the Far East. It can be boiled like spinach or blanched and served as a salad.

Silverweed

SCIENTIFIC NAME: *Potentilla anserina* (also *Argentina anserina*).

OTHER POPULAR NAMES: Goose grass, silver cinquefoil, cramp weed, goose tansy, moor grass.

FAMILY: Rosaceae—Rose Family.

RANGE: Silverweed grows on wet, clayey soil in meadows, along stream beds and ditches, and in pastures. It is widely distributed throughout the world.

DESCRIPTION: From the root-stock emerge bundles of leaves and many runners which fasten themselves to the soil again and cast out new roots. The pinnate leaves are sharp and toothed and have on their undersides tiny hairs that gleam silver-white. The inflorescences rise up leaflets from the runners and bear large flowers of gleaming, golden yellow.

ELEMENTS CONTAINED: Tannin, sugar, mucilage.

MEDICINAL USE: The plant—*Herba Potentillae anserinae*; the root —*Radix Potentillae anserinae*; the international designation is *Herba* or *Radix Anserinae*.

Kneipp gave a few grains of silverweed scalded in hot milk when symptoms of his patients became noticeable, indicating the approach of cramps. He recommended the plant especially for women attacked by cramps. Folk medicine also made use of the plant in affectations of the mucous membrane of the digestive tract, in cases of colic, asthma and whooping cough. These internal uses were made with a tea consisting of 1–4 grams (15.4–61.6 grains avdp) scalded by pouring 1 cup boiling water over it. In modern medicine, the medicinal effect is disputed.

CULINARY USE: The roots, which taste like parsnips, can be eaten raw, roasted or boiled, and were once dried and ground to make a kind of meal.

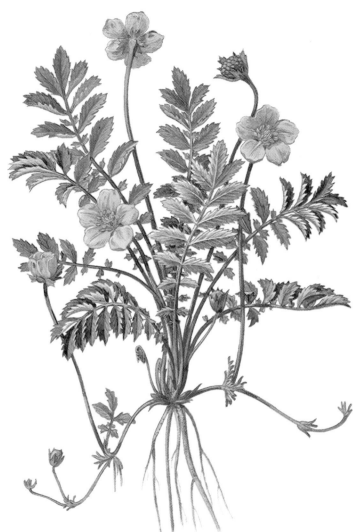

Silverweed

Solomon's Seal

SOLOMON'S SEAL

SCIENTIFIC NAMES: *Polygonatum officinale (Convallaria polygonatum, Convallaria multiflora).*

OTHER POPULAR NAME: Angular Solomon's seal.

FAMILY: Liliaceae—Lily Family.

RANGE: Found in Europe and Asia in light, dry places in both deciduous and conifer forests and at the edge of woods, *C. multiflora* is found throughout the United States and Canada.

DESCRIPTION: If provided with the traces of shoots from previous years, the thick, white root-stock creeps horizontally. Out of it sprouts the stalk in a graceful arc, with numerous oval, pointed leaves developing in rhythmic order. From the leaf axes, which occur both in pairs and singly, droop greenish-white little bells on long stems. Blue fruits as large as wild plums decorate the plant.

ELEMENTS CONTAINED: Mucilage, asparagine, convallaria-glycosides.

MEDICINAL USE: The root—*Radix Sigilli Salomonis.*

The effect of Solomon's seal extends to the regeneration processes in contusions, hematomas, and skin inflation, to diabetes and diuresis (increased excretion of urine).

CULINARY USE: None.

GARDEN SORREL

SCIENTIFIC NAME: *Rumex acetosa.*

OTHER POPULAR NAMES: Dock, sorrel, common sorrel.

FAMILY: Polygonaceae—Buckwheat or Knotweed Family.

RANGE: Garden sorrel grows everywhere in Central Europe on wet meadows and fields, along roadsides and slopes. It is naturalized in North America. One of the principal cultivated forms is Large Belleville.

DESCRIPTION: The arrowhead-shaped, glossy leaves grow from a thin, perpendicular root. The stem is scantily clad with leaves that grow smaller toward the top bearing the reddish, shimmering flower panicles, which, when sorrel grows in large quantity, gives the meadow a reddish shimmer. The plant is wind-pollinated.

ELEMENTS CONTAINED: Oxalic acid, a small amount of a bitter principle and tannin.

MEDICINAL USE: The plant—*Herba Rumex acetosae*; the seeds—*Semen Rumex acetosae*.

The leaves of the sorrel plant were used in folk medicine mainly for blood cleansing in the spring cure. The seeds are a popular folk remedy for worms in children. Take 1–2 grams (15.4–30.8 grains avdp) of the seeds and scald them with a cup of boiling water.

CULINARY USE: In many areas, the leaves of the sorrel are eaten in salad or prepared as a soup, and are used to give a zest to vinegar. Sorrel may also be braised or puréed. Fresh sorrel may be frozen.

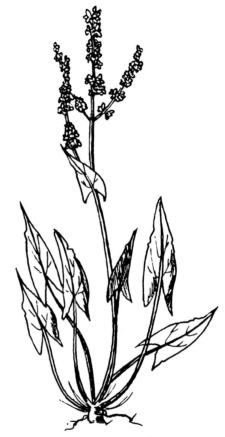

Garden Sorrel

WILD STRAWBERRY

SCIENTIFIC NAME: *Fragaria vesca* (also *F. alpina*).

OTHER POPULAR NAMES: Wood strawberry, hautboy.

FAMILY: Rosaceae—Rose Family.

RANGE: Wild strawberries are widespread in North America, Europe and many other parts of the world, in sunny glades in the forests.

DESCRIPTION: Most people are familiar with the little wild strawberry, which thrusts its white flower heads out of the grass on slopes, at the edge of the woods, in clearings and among new plantations of young trees. In former times, people ascribed to the wild strawberry all kinds of powers against demons and they not only used the berries for food but also as a medicinal plant.

ELEMENTS CONTAINED: The plant contains tannin, some mucilage, sugar and acids. The berries are rich in minerals, such as iron, sodium, potassium, calcium, and phosphorus. They have an abundant surplus of alkali and a lot of vitamin C.

MEDICINAL USE: The plant—*Herba Fragariae*; the fruit—*Fructus Fragariae*.

A tea (1 teaspoonful of the leaves, scalded by pouring 1 cup of boiling water over it) is given to children for slight cases of diarrhea and is also recommended for jaundice. The tea is exceptionally good as a blood purifier and a diuretic.

The botanist Linnaeus writes that he cured his gout with fresh wild strawberries, which can probably be attributed to their abundance of alkali. Strawberries as dessert in cases of ordinary undernourishment provide a good means of restoring balance owing to their large content of minerals and vitamin C. They are also given patients in cases of circulatory trouble, nervous weakness and in cases of kidney and bladder trouble.

CULINARY USE: Wherever wild strawberries grow in abundance, picnickers enlarge their open-air meal with these tiny, extra-sweet berries. They are so small that a great many must be picked to provide a suitable dessert for one person.

Wild Strawberry

Sundew

SCIENTIFIC NAME: *Drosera rotundifolia.*

OTHER POPULAR NAMES: Round-leaved sundew, common sundew.

FAMILY: Droseraceae—Sundew Family.

RANGE: In North America, northern and central Europe, sundew grows on peat-soil, swampy meadows, and around the edges of marshy lakes and ponds, deeply embedded in sphagnum moss. It is found in moist sandy and peaty soil in Canada and the United States.

DESCRIPTION: There occur in Europe three insectivorous *Drosera* species. In addition to *Drosera rotundifolia*, there are *Drosera intermedia* and *Drosera longifolia* (long-leaved). Out of a rosette of long-stemmed leaves climbs a flower spike with small, white star-flowers on it, which open only at midday. The most interesting part of this plant is the leaves. On the long stems are thickened leaf-ends, which are stuck with reddish glandular hairs, like a pincushion. The hairs are thickened at their tips and discharge a clear, sticky sap. The drops twinkle like diamonds on the ends of the hairs in the sun, but this sap is full of danger. If a curious insect alights upon the leaf, it remains stuck to the hairs. The hairs have only been waiting for this stimulus. They bend downward, enclosing the tiny prisoner, and digest it with the enzyme and an acid. Both are contained in the glandular sap.

After this occurrence, the leaves open up again and one sees only the indigestible remains of the insect, such as the legs and the wings. The sundew is dependent on such nourishment, because the roots are not sufficiently developed. This state of affairs may appear distasteful to many, and yet, this "unnaturalness" is quite normal. The deficient root structure gives the sundew somewhat the aspect of an animal. It almost seems not to be attached to the ground.

Yet, this state of affairs is found to exist to some degree in many other flowering plants that are pollinated by insects. Some flowers take in nectar-seeking insects, enfold them, hold them prisoner a moment, and then release them again. It is a matter of give and take. The flowers give their nectar, the insects bring pollen for the fructification. The animals eat the plants and give their excrement as fertilizer for the plants. The plants take in carbon dioxide which the animals give off, and give off oxygen, which the animals require to breathe. These relationships between

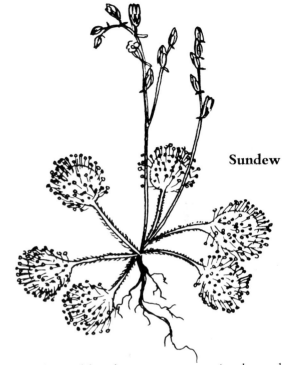

Sundew

the plant and animal kingdoms are very extensive, but such a discussion would go far beyond the limits of this book.

ELEMENTS CONTAINED: The sundew contains one of the pepsin-like enzymes, which digests albumen, and, in addition, organic acids—citric, formic, acetic, and malic—as well as some essential oil.

MEDICINAL USE: The plant—*Herba Droserae rotundifoliae, Herba Rorellae, Herba Roris Solis.*

In the 13th century, alchemists prepared a remedy from sundew, with which beneficial results were obtained against consumption (phthisis). Later, in the 18th century, herbals contained information treating this subject. Today, sundew is used in cases of whooping cough, asthma, morning sickness of pregnant women, and as a stomachic with 1 gram (15.4 grains avdp) scalded with 2 cupfuls of boiling water. Larger amounts have an injurious effect. Sundew sap causes milk to curdle.

CULINARY USE: The leaves of the sundew may be eaten raw in salads or cooked like spinach.

SWEET FLAG

SCIENTIFIC NAME: *Acorus calamus*.

OTHER POPULAR NAMES: Sweet grass, sweet cane, sweet sedge, calmus, calamus, myrtle flag, sweet root, sweet rush.

FAMILY: Araceae (sometimes called Aroideae)—Arum Family.

RANGE: Sweet flag hails from the Orient; in the 16th century it was brought to Vienna by the Turks. It has since become widespread in Europe and grows on river banks, pond edges, and along streams and ditches. It is just as much at home in swampy regions of the lowlands as it is in the mountains, up to an altitude of 1,100 metres (3,630 feet). Common to the northern hemisphere, it grows on the borders of ponds and marshes throughout the United States.

DESCRIPTION: This water plant has a fleshy, creeping root-stock in the mud. The root has a spicy scent. Its broad, erect, linear leaves grow to a metre (40 inches) in length and reach out over the surface of the water. From the side of the pistils, which look a great deal like the leaves, a somewhat crooked spike, 4–6 cm ($1\frac{5}{8}$–$2\frac{3}{8}$ inches) long, studded with small, greenish blossoms, bursts forth in June. In front of the 6 green sheaths constituting the calyx are located the stamens with yellow sac and double to triple ovaries (seed buds). The juiceless, also greenish, berries seldom succeed in ripening.

ELEMENTS CONTAINED: 1.5–5 per cent essential oil, a bitter principle, methyl amine, choline, tannin, mucilage.

MEDICINAL USE: Root-stock—*Rhizoma Calami*; oil—*Oleum Calami*.

Externally, the thinned root extract finds a broad area of use as a mouthwash in gum troubles, such as inflamed or bleeding gums, in cases of toothache, and as a bath additive for children with scrofula or rickets, particularly with curvature of the bones. Calamus oil (sweet flag oil) is used to rub on sickly children.

In cases of excessive stomach acidity and fermentation or septic processes in the intestines, 1–4 grams (15.4–61.6 grains avdp) of the finely chopped calamus root are scalded with boiling water, or briefly boiled.

CULINARY USE: Since calamus root is exceptionally good as bitters, it is given as an appetite stimulant.

The root-stock can be candied.

Sweet Flag

COMMON TANSY

SCIENTIFIC NAME: *Tanacetum vulgare.*

OTHER POPULAR NAMES: Wild tansy, buttons, alecost, wild agrimony, goose grass, bitter buttons, parsley fern, tansy.

FAMILY: Compositae—Composite Family.

RANGE: Common tansy grows in Europe in regions of moist, warm climate, in the banks of the great river valleys, along roadsides, field borders, along ditches and on slopes. It was carried from Europe to America.

DESCRIPTION: This plant prefers sandy-loam soils. As it thrusts its sturdy stalk with broad, pinnate leaves out of its blackish-brown root-stock, it looks similar to the ferns, but when it grows to metre height (40 inches), it radiates its stem toward all sides, and on the end of each stemlet sits the little golden flower. Since the little flower heads consist only of tube-flowers, they really look like buttons. The strong, sharp smell of the leaves and blossoms gave the plant in folk-talk the name of stink fern, among others.

ELEMENTS CONTAINED: Essential oil, which contains up to 70 per cent thujone, a bitter principle, a small quantity of tannin, various acids.

MEDICINAL USE: The leaves—*Folia Tanaceti*; blossoms—*Flores Tanaceti*; leaves and blossoms—*Herba Tanaceti*; seeds—*Semen Tanaceti.*

Common tansy is a well known worming agent, the special effect of which extends to ascarides (intestinal worms) and maggots. Taken in small doses, it helps in cases of slight disturbance of the digestive tract. This medicinal plant should only be used after consultation with a physician, because the essential oil unleashes poisonous phenomena, which can even lead to a fatal outcome. In taking measures against intestinal worms and maggots, it is better for this reason to use the wild carrot.

CULINARY USE: Tansy was used at one time to give a tang to puddings and pancakes.

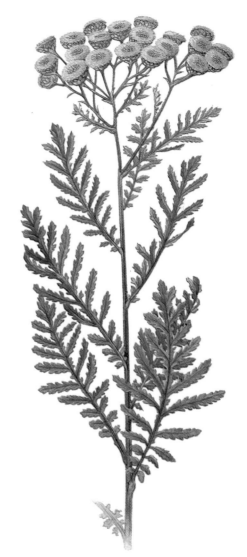

Common Tansy

TARRAGON

SCIENTIFIC NAME: *Artemisia dracunculus.*

OTHER POPULAR NAME: Estragon.

FAMILY: Compositae—Composite Family.

RANGE: Tarragon originated in eastern Europe and northern Asia, and is cultivated in many other parts of the world.

DESCRIPTION: Tarragon is a shrubby plant about 2 feet (60 cm) high, with dense foliage and ridged, somewhat woody stem and branches. The alternate leaves are narrow, pointed at the tip and undivided. The brownish root is gnarled, but not woody. The tiny greenish-white flowers, borne in panicles, bloom in midsummer. When the leaves are crushed, they give off a scent similar to anise.

ELEMENTS CONTAINED: Essential oil.

MEDICINAL USE: The oil (extracted from the green parts of the plant) is used to stimulate appetite and as a diuretic.

CULINARY USE: Tarragon is widely used to add zest to vinegar, and in fish sauces, mayonnaise and stock, and is an essential ingredient of sauce Béarnaise. Tarragon should be used cautiously in salads and stews, as it does not blend well with many other herbal seasonings. It can be used fresh or dried. Fresh tarragon leaves are a must in the French dish *oeufs en gelée* (eggs in aspic).

Tarragon

Blessed Thistle

SCIENTIFIC NAMES: *Cnicus benedictus (Carduus benedictus, Centaurea benedicta).*

OTHER POPULAR NAMES: St. Benedict's thistle, holy thistle.

FAMILY: Compositae—Composite Family.

RANGE: Native to the Mediterranean region, the blessed thistle was carried over the Alps during the Middle Ages and cultivated in gardens as a medicinal plant.

DESCRIPTION: This annual plant grows about knee-high. The yellowish flower heads barely appear among the long leaves edged with sharp points and bristling with spines.

ELEMENTS CONTAINED: Glycosidic bitter principle (cnicin), tannic acid, some essential oil, resin, a great deal of mucilage, potassium, calcium, magnesium salts.

MEDICINAL USE: The plant—*Herba Cardui benedicti.* An extract *(Extractum Cardui benedicti)* is pressed from the plant after it has had hot water poured over it.

Cnicus benedictus used to be applied externally as a healing agent for wounds and burns.

Modern medicine prefers internal use; 2–5 grams (30.8–77 grains avdp) are scalded by pouring 1 cup of boiling water over the plant. Its main effect is to benefit the physiological pepsin exchange (the stomach, intestines, liver and gall bladder), as well as the mucous membranes of the breathing apparatus.

CULINARY USE: None.

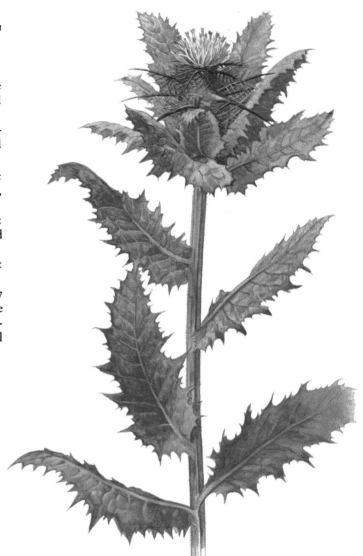

Blessed Thistle

Thyme

THYME

SCIENTIFIC NAME: *Thymus vulgaris.*

OTHER POPULAR NAMES: Garden thyme, common thyme.

FAMILY: Labiatae—Mint Family.

RANGE: The primary habitat of thyme is on the stony slopes of the Mediterranean region. In Europe and America, it is cultivated in gardens as a kitchen herb.

DESCRIPTION: The unassuming thyme plants, which appear from the ground in thick, pink to semi-violet cushions, seem to grow right out of the naked, native rock and to have no need for water. It is true, this labiate lives almost entirely on cosmic sources, on sun and warmth. The narrow, fleshy little leaves stand opposed on the stem reaching eagerly upward. The blossoms have a sharp aroma and are sought after by bees. In Germany, thyme received the popular name of bee herb.

ELEMENTS CONTAINED: Essential oil, which contains up to 50 per cent thymol (thyme camphor or thymic acid), saponin, resin, a bitter principle and tannin.

MEDICINAL USE: The blooming plant—*Herba Thymi*; oil—*Oleum Thymi*; thymic acid—*thymol*.

It is used externally in baths for treating children with rickets or scrofula. Internal use, however, is more important in respect to chronic bronchial catarrh, whooping cough, and especially with regard to coughs, for thyme loosens the mucus and has a sedative effect on irritations of the air passages. It is also an anti-spasmodic and is effective against gastritis, stomach spasms and colic, by reason of its regulation of heat processes in these areas. It is said to promote digestion.

CULINARY USE: Has a spicy aroma and a slightly biting taste. Fresh: Use the finely chopped leaves. Dried: Use the whole leaf, powdered or ground. It is popular in soups, especially clam chowder, and can add seasoning to chopped meat, liver and dumplings, marrow-balls, turkey stuffing, meat, game, and fowl dishes, fish, herb butter, sauces or gravies, legumes, stews, as well as in pickling, marinades, and in the production of liqueurs.

Keep in a tightly closed container, away from air and light.

CREEPING THYME

SCIENTIFIC NAME: *Thymus serpyllum.*

OTHER POPULAR NAMES: Mother of thyme, wild thyme, wild caraway.

FAMILY: Labiatae—Mint Family.

RANGE: Creeping thyme grows especially on sunny, dew-damp mountain meadows and slopes on the southern and northern faces of the Alps and, in addition, in central Europe. It has been naturalized in the United States.

DESCRIPTION: The sweet-scented plant decorates the mountain slopes from May into September with its decumbent branches, small, opposed leaves, and the richly blooming flower heads of reddish blossoms.

ELEMENTS CONTAINED: Essential oil, some thymol, carvacrol.

MEDICINAL USE: The blooming plant—*Herba Thymi serpylli cum Floribus*; or, *Herba Serpylli.*

In folk medicine, creeping thyme was applied as a "women's herb." A tea of creeping thyme was given pregnant women and it was also called menstruation-promoting. Creeping thyme is given nowadays for disturbances of the digestion. Its antispasmodic effect is corroborated in cases of stomach cramps, asthma, epilepsy, and colic. Tea is made from 2–4 grams (30.8–61.6 grains avdp) of the plant scalded with 1 cup of boiling water.

External use as an addition to baths for scrofulous and sickly children is commonly known.

CULINARY USE: None.

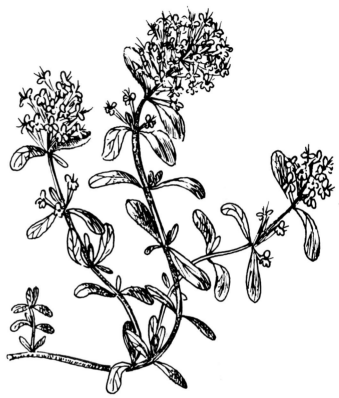

Creeping Thyme

Toadflax

TOADFLAX

SCIENTIFIC NAME: *Linaria vulgaris.*

OTHER POPULAR NAMES: Common toadflax, butter and eggs, yellow toadflax, wild flax, common linaria, snapdragon.

FAMILY: Scrophulariaceae—Figwort Family.

RANGE: Toadflax grows everywhere in Europe on meadows, along roadsides, on refuse dumps, stony fields, slopes, and at the edge of woods, and is naturalized in the United States.

DESCRIPTION: Toadflax has nothing whatever to do with flax *(Linum usitatissimum).* It got its name solely because women in the Middle Ages prepared a decoction from the plant with alum, which they applied to their linens as starch. Since the use of blueing was not to be discovered for a long time yet, they gave their linens a yellow tint, which was produced with toadflax, mignonette, dyer's broom, or saffron.

This widespread plant has narrow, lanceolate leaves and is especially conspicuous owing to its large, yellow, compressed spur-flowers, which exhibit 5-pointed blossoms with 5 stamens and a 2- to 4-fold ovary (seed bud).

ELEMENTS CONTAINED: Glycosides, among them linarin, organic acids such as formic, tannic, citric, and malic; gum, sugar, and pectin.

MEDICINAL USE: The blooming plant—*Herba Linariae cum floribus.*

Formerly, toadflax was used as a diuretic and purging agent. It is hardly used at all today. Since animals will not eat it, it can be used in stalls as straw for driving out vermin. In many places, toadflax is boiled in milk and the decoction is used as a fly poison.

CULINARY USE: None.

Tormentil

SCIENTIFIC NAMES: *Potentilla erecta (P. recta, P. tormentilla).*
OTHER POPULAR NAMES: Cinquefoil, blood root.
FAMILY: Rosaceae—Rose Family.
RANGE: In Europe and Asia, tormentil grows practically everywhere in damp woods and along the edges of meadows.
DESCRIPTION: The sturdy, finger-thick root-stock is the principal organ of this plant. What peers out of the soil of damp meadowland are the small, 4-petalled, yellow flowers, among which are first discovered the 3- to 5-fingered leaflets which, in the tormentil, show in addition two spectacularly large, serrated floral leaves.
ELEMENTS CONTAINED: 17–20 per cent tannic acid, a dyestuff (tormentilla red), quinovic acid, ellagic acid, traces of essential oil, resin, gum, starch and calcium oxalate.
MEDICINAL USE: The root-stock—*Rhizoma Tormentillae.*

A decoction made from 2–3 grams (30.8–46.2 grains avdp) briefly boiled in 1 cup of water, is used externally against inflammation of the mucous membrane of the mouth, inflammation of the gums, and catarrh of the mouth and throat (pharyngitis), as a gargle, as well as in compresses used on skin wounds, weeping or dry eczema, and herpetic skin eruptions.

The region of internal use is, in particular, the digestive tract. Bleeding, persistent diarrhea, inflammations, and catarrhs are also beneficially influenced.

CULINARY USE: None.

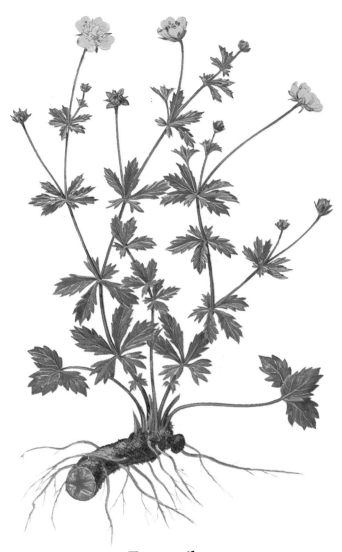

Tormentil

Valerian

SCIENTIFIC NAME: *Valeriana officinalis.*

OTHER POPULAR NAMES: Common valerian, garden heliotrope, great wild valerian, fragrant valerian, vandal root, English valerian, setwall, phu, setewale, capon's tail, all-heal, St. George's herb.

FAMILY: Valerianaceae—Valerian Family.

RANGE: Valerian grows throughout Central Europe on mountain slopes, meadows, in woods, and on the banks of streams. It is also found in northern Asia and has been naturalized in North America.

DESCRIPTION: Even in ancient times, valerian had a particularly good reputation as a medicinal plant. The ancient Germans called it *Velandsurt* (Wieland's root) after Wayland the Smith, a folk hero. The Serbs call it *odaljan* (from *odoljeti* = to conquer). Among them, it is even commemorated in a song, in which women are advised not to neglect the precious herb but to wear it always in their waistband.

Common valerian *(Valeriana officinalis)* has pinnate leaves on its tubular stem, which grows to a height of about 70 cm ($27\frac{1}{2}$ inches), and at the top a flower cluster called a cyme. Cats are attracted to valerian—they give a loud cry when they encounter it and soon fall into a state of downright ecstasy.

ELEMENTS CONTAINED: Valerian oil, which has several components, among which is included isovaleric acid bornyl ester, to which the calming effect of valerian is ascribed. Valerian also contains mucilage, sugar, gum, tannic acid, resin, lipase, oxidase, and malic, formic, and acetic acids.

MEDICINAL USE: The root—*Radix Valerianae.*

Valerian is used externally only for nervous eye-trouble, weakness of the eyes, and eye-strain.

Internal use, however, is highly regarded for its effectiveness in treating nervousness, nervous insomnia, conditions of anxiety, states of nervous convulsion, nervous vertigo, and coughs, as well as nervous complaints connected with menopause. Dosage is 10–30 drops of the tincture in some water, or 1 teaspoonful of the finely chopped root in $\frac{1}{4}$ litre (about $8\frac{1}{2}$ oz) of water. Allow the tea to boil for a bit, then steep for 5 minutes before straining.

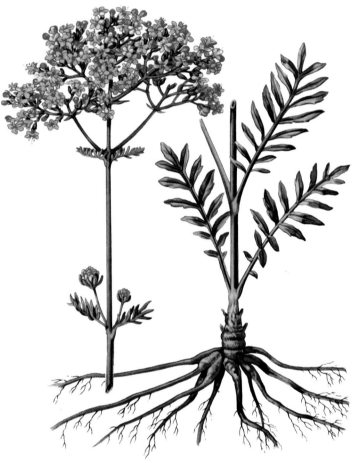

Valerian

CULINARY USE: A native American valerian, *V. edulis*, found widely west of the Appalachian Mountains, was prized by the American Indians for its carrot-like root, which they baked.

Veronica

SCIENTIFIC NAME: *Veronica officinalis.*

OTHER POPULAR NAMES: Speedwell, Paul's betony, ground-hele, fluellin (also fluellen), low speedwell.

FAMILY: Scrophulariaceae—Figwort Family.

RANGE: Veronica grows practically everywhere in Europe, Asia and North America, in dry soils (on slopes, pastures, and in open conifer forests).

DESCRIPTION: Common veronica has a hairy stem that creeps along the ground with equally hairy, opposed leaves. Out of their angles sprout the bright blue flower clusters. The terminal shoot of practically all species of veronica bears no flowers.

ELEMENTS CONTAINED: A bitter principle, tannin, essential oil, saponin.

MEDICINAL USE: The whole plant—*Herba Veronicae.*

Veronica tea is made from 3–4 grams (46.2–61.6 grains avdp) scalded by pouring on 1 cup of boiling water and straining after standing 5 minutes; it has always been dispensed in folk medicine as a universal remedy for liver, stomach and intestinal troubles, as well as recommended in cases of rheumatism, gout, bronchitis and cystitis. The freshly squeezed juice of the veronica plant is recommended for skin troubles.

CULINARY USE: None.

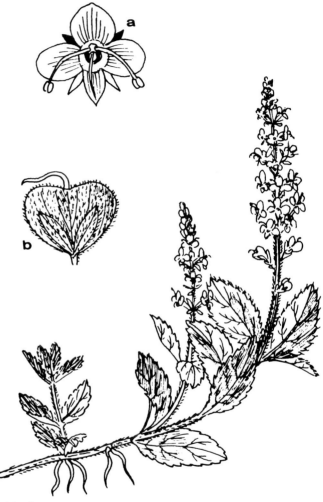

(a) Flower
(b) Capsule

Veronica

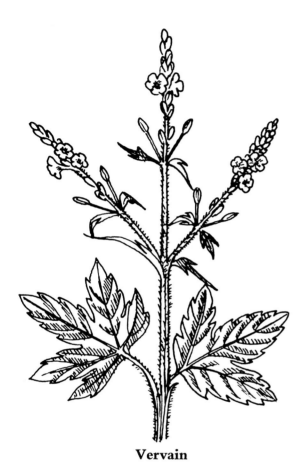

Vervain

VERVAIN

SCIENTIFIC NAME: *Verbena officinalis.*

OTHER POPULAR NAMES: Verbena, vervein.

FAMILY: Verbenaceae—Vervain Family.

RANGE: Vervain grows throughout Europe, along roads, walls and fences, and preferably in villages. It is native to Europe and Asia but has escaped to America, where it grows as a weed. It is sometimes cultivated.

DESCRIPTION: In the autumn, a strange and unpretentious plant grows among other herbage along village fences—this is vervain. It stands stiffly erect to a height of 30–60 cm (1–2 feet). It has opposed, three-lobed, toothed leaves and small, lilac-hued blossoms on thin, equally erect spikes which are formed at the ends of the main stem and of the equally stiff side branches.

The Druids believed the plant to have magical powers, though this meaning is lost today. Vervain has flowers that are very like those of labiate plants (Mint Family); yet, under closer scrutiny, the difference is readily seen. The style of the pistil does not separate the seed compartments from each other until it has risen from their top.

ELEMENTS CONTAINED: A bitter principle, a tannin that turns iron green, glycoside, verbenalin, invertin (invertase), emulin and mucilage.

MEDICINAL USE: The plant—*Herba Verbenae.*

In ancient times, vervain was a universal remedy. Today it is used as a diuretic and diaphoretic (sudorific) in rheumatism and chronic bronchitis. Old-time herbals recommend it for migraine, since it regulates the activity of those large, secretionary organs, the liver and the kidneys. Two teaspoons of the dried herb added to $\frac{1}{2}$ litre (1 pint) of boiling water makes an infusion which should be drunk cold.

CULINARY USE: Popular as a tea, especially in Europe. Can be made strong or weak. A related plant, lemon verbena *(Lippia citriodora),* native to Peru and Chile, has been naturalized in southern Europe and India, but is not hardy in cooler climates. The leaves are used to give a lemony taste to cold drinks.

Sweet Violet

SCIENTIFIC NAME: *Viola odorata.*

OTHER POPULAR NAMES: Wild violet, garden violet, florists' violet.

FAMILY: Violaceae—Violet Family.

RANGE: Violets grow practically everywhere in temperate regions, along fences, hedges and the edges of woods.

DESCRIPTION: The Greeks dedicated this beautiful spring flower to the goddess Persephone, which, as a symbol of the immortal soul of the plant world, causes perpetual revival. The many-branched root–stock that forms a nest of old stems and leaves, prepares a rosette of saw-toothed, heart-shaped leaves in a shade of green that harmonizes with the blue, sweet-smelling flowers. In addition, runners contribute to maintaining the tender blossoms in spring storms and cold. They hang in filaments out of the rosette, touch the ground, and grow new roots, leaves and blossoms.

ELEMENTS CONTAINED: The blossoms contain salicyclic acid, blue dyestuff and essential oil; the roots contain an alkaloid (violine = viola-emetine); in all parts, albumen, mucilage, sugar, and gum.

MEDICINAL USE: The leaves—*Folia Violae odoratae*; flowers—*Flores Violae odoratae*; plant—*Herba Violae odoratae*; root—*Radix Violae odoratae*.

Violet tea made from 2–4 grams (30.8–61.6 grains avdp) scalded with 1 cup of boiling water, is used externally as a superior gargle for sore throat, difficulty in swallowing, and inflammatory changes in the mouth.

Internally, the tea performs good service in whooping cough, coughs, bronchial catarrh, and in cases of mucous blockage of the air passages. The light decotion of 2–4 grams (30.8–61.6 grains avdp) of the root induces vomiting.

CULINARY USE: Whole violet blossoms are candied and used in confectionery to decorate cakes and desserts, especially in Europe. They can also be eaten as candies. In France a liqueur, *ratafia de violettes*, is distilled from the petals.

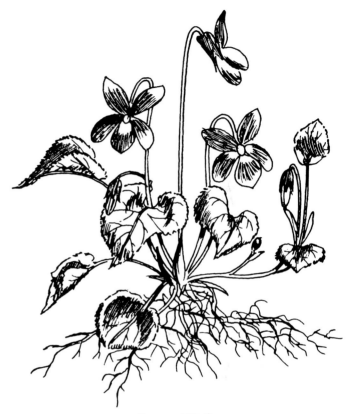

Sweet Violet

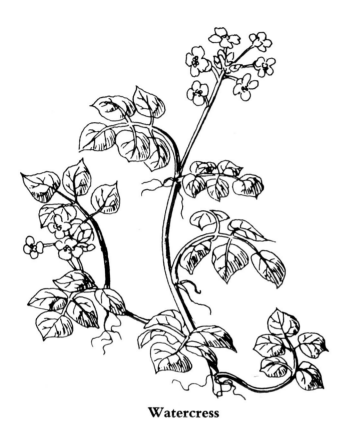

Watercress

WATERCRESS

SCIENTIFIC NAMES: *Nasturtium officinale* (*Roripa nasturtium aquaticum*, *Radicula nasturtium aquaticum*.)

OTHER POPULAR NAME: Tall nasturtium.

FAMILY: Cruciferae—Mustard Family.

RANGE: Throughout Europe, watercress is found in clear streams, on flat banks, by springs and in wet meadows. Whole plots of watercress can grow under a full metre (40 inches) of water. This plant has been widely naturalized in North America.

DESCRIPTION: This plant of leaves and sprouts develops from leaf node to leaf node, flowing along, so to speak, with the water. Annual growth starts when there is no longer ice in the streams, but snow still lies upon the fields. The leaves are in the shape of rounded ovals made up of pinnae (leaflets). In early summer, the plant produces loose clusters of flowers, the white blossoms of which are self-pollinating.

ELEMENTS CONTAINED: Sulphurous essential oil, oil of mustard, glycosides, a bitter principle, abundant vitamin C, some iodine.

MEDICINAL USE: The plant—*Herba Nasturtii*.

Watercress is used principally as a spring tonic, for regulating the metabolism and the flow of bile, for tightening up loose teeth, as well as in cases of rheumatism, eczema and acne; and as a diuretic agent.

CULINARY USE: One way to use watercress is to add it to a salad, or chop the plant fine and mix it in with a salad. Its whole leaves and stems are also eaten in tea sandwiches and used as a garnish on steaks and chops. Watercress is a spicy addition to cream soups, or can be made as the Chinese and Japanese do into a clear soup. It may also be cooked in the same manner as spinach, puréed with potatoes, or simmered in butter.

SWEET WOODRUFF

SCIENTIFIC NAME: *Asperula odorata.*

OTHER POPULAR NAMES: Woodruff, master of the woods.

FAMILY: Rubiaceae—Madder Family.

RANGE: This charming plant grows throughout Europe and northern Asia, especially in light beech woods, occasionally also in fir forests, and has been naturalized in parts of eastern North America.

DESCRIPTION: Woodruff grows among dead leaves, under the light-green of the beeches. It stands stiffly erect, forming leaf-whorl after leaf-whorl, topping off with a false-umbel of little white star-shaped flowers. Its scent, which comes from cumarin glycoside, does not become strong until the plant begins to die away on completion of its flowering cycle.

ELEMENTS CONTAINED: Cumarin, tannin, a bitter principle, citric acid, and catechuic acid (catechin).

MEDICINAL USE: The entire plant when in flower—*Herba Asperulae,* or *Herba Matrisilvae.*

Woodruff tea made from 2–4 grams (30.8–61.6 grains avdp) scalded with 1 cup of boiling water, has a stimulating effect on the metabolism and a moderately diuretic action. Woodruff is a prized remedy for kidney and bladder troubles, especially for obstructions, and gravel and stone troubles, in cases of dropsy, liver congestion and back pressure (or stoppage) in the gall bladder and, not least, in cases of insomnia.

CULINARY USE: Woodruff is used in making certain wines, especially in Germany, where it forms an ingredient of May wine.

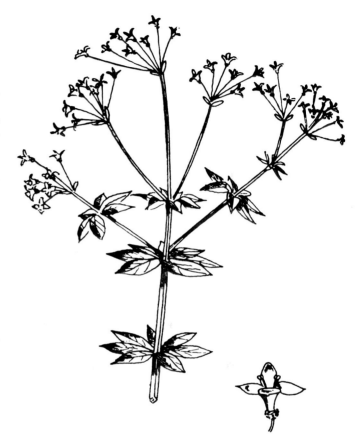

Sweet Woodruff

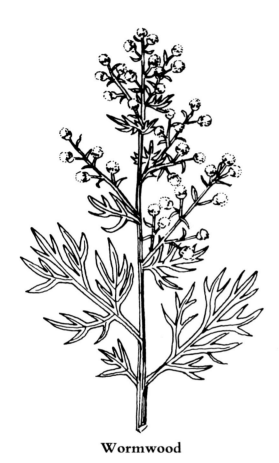

Wormwood

Wormwood

SCIENTIFIC NAME: *Artemisia absinthium*.

OTHER POPULAR NAMES: Common wormwood, absinthium, absinthe.

FAMILY: Compositae—Composite Family.

RANGE: Even the ancient Egyptians were acquainted with wormwood and used it as a medicinal plant, also in their religious rites. The Greeks and Romans held it in the same esteem, while we today find it just as well known as a medicinal plant. It is written in an old herbal: "Wormwood is an unrivaled herb, kept by the ancients and excellently used in religious services and triumphs." It is native to the warm, Mediterranean countries, but today it grows wild over all of Eurasia in nitrogen-rich, stony and hence loose, soil.

DESCRIPTION: The perennial root-stock of this stately subshrub puts forth many shoots with silvery-green, abundantly pinnate leaves, which in midsummer bear loose clusters of yellow umbels on erect panicles.

ELEMENTS CONTAINED: Essential oils contained in it are: thujone, thujyl alcohol, pinene, azulene, and phellanden; a bitter principle, glycoside (absinthin and anabsinthin); tannin, resin, vitamins (C and B_6), and, in the ashes, nitric and silicic acids.

MEDICINAL USE: The plant—*Herba Absinthii*.

Wormwood is used especially for the digestive tract. It eliminates pressure on the stomach, a feeling of fullness, loss of appetite, heartburn, too much or too little stomach acid, gas-formation in stomach and bowels, and congestion of the liver or gall bladder. Continued use of wormwood, however, is not advisable, since the essential oil is poisonous and can lead to injury. The regular use of absinthe, to which wormwood's essential oil has been added, has a damaging effect on the reproductive organs.

CULINARY USE: As an alcoholic liquor, absinthe is so intoxicating its manufacture has been banned almost everywhere.

Yarrow

SCIENTIFIC NAME: *Achillea millifolium.*

OTHER POPULAR NAMES: Milfoil, millefoil, thousand seal, nosebleed, common yarrow.

FAMILY: Compositae—Composite Family.

RANGE: Yarrow is widespread in the northern hemisphere and grows in meadows and pastures, along field borders, roadsides, fields and on the edges of woods.

DESCRIPTION: In early spring, tender, bright green, pinnate leaves appear at the base of the withered plant of the previous year, which still stands there, stiff and brown. The stem grows wiry and strong, bringing forth node after node, leaf after leaf, until the sun finally reaches its highest position in the sky for the year. Then the stalk spreads out in fine branches and forms a horizontal terminal, the false umbel, with small, white, often pinkly shimmering flowers.

ELEMENTS CONTAINED: Blue-green essential oil with azulene and cineole content; a bitter principle achileine, tannin, aconitic acid, resin, inulin, asparagine, gum, acetic and malic acids, silicic acid, an exceptional quantity of potassium, sulphur.

MEDICINAL USE: The plant—*Herba Millifolii*; blooming plant—*Herba Millifolii cum Floribus*; flowers—*Flores Millifolii.*

Yarrow stimulates the metabolism, aids the stomach, promotes appetite, stimulates liver action and blood building. It promotes the healing of wounds and has an antispasmodic and anodyne (pain-killing) effect in colics. In cases of irregular menses and during the menopause, this popular medicinal plant is used as a decoction. Make with 2–4 grams (30.8–61.6 grains avdp) and scald with 1 cup of boiling water, but never boil.

CULINARY USE: In some countries yarrow is used instead of hops to give sharpness to beer.

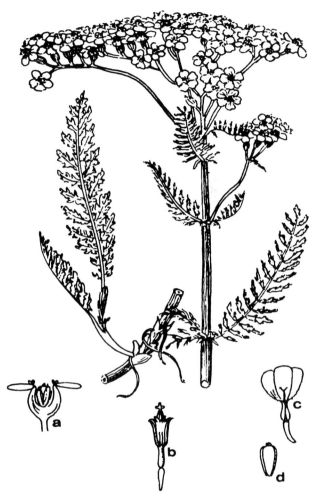

(a) Cross-section of small flower head
(b) Disc floret
(c) Ray flower
(d) Fruit

Yarrow

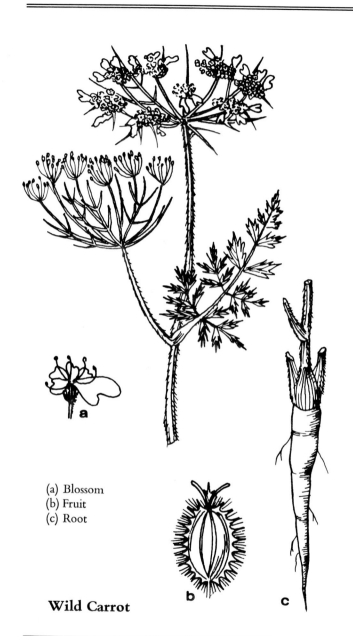

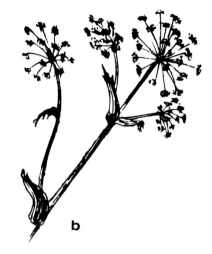

(a) Fruit
(b) Flowers

Angelica

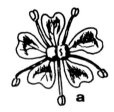

(a) Flower
(b) Fruit

(a) Blossom
(b) Fruit
(c) Root

Wild Carrot

**Poison
Hemlock**

GENERAL INDEX

SCIENTIFIC NAME INDEX

POPULAR NAME INDEX

GEOGRAPHICAL INDEX